HOW TO BE GLUTEN FREE AND KEEP YOUR FRIENDS

Recipes by Anna Barnett

Additional text by Quadrille

PHOTOGRAPHY BY KIM LIGHTBODY

Hardie Grant

QUADRILLE

Gluten-free/dom

///

Living gluten-free can feel like a massive life obstacle and, let's face it, a little bit like a punishment — like being handcuffed in a room full of fluffy puppies or blindfolded in the face of a life-changing sunset.

If you're new to the gluten-free game, you'll wonder how you're ever going to survive / smile again / stop complaining / enjoy yourself at any event or outing ever, ever, ever. If you're a gluten-free pro and haven't been near a cinnamon bun in as long as you can remember, then, firstly, bravo! And secondly, you might be very bored of all your tried-and-tested recipes and methods for navigating life as a gluten-free diner. Either way, this book is here to help!

It's packed with exciting, globally-inspired recipes that will awaken your taste buds and make you forget you ever wanted a dull bread roll. It's also awash with tips and tricks for living a more friend-friendly gluten-free existence, from knowing which flour will help you make that towering celebration cake for your sceptical flatmate, to ordering food in a restaurant without feeling angry / sad / embarrassed.

Use this book to inspire you to experiment with food and flavours and to feel more confident and excited to move forward on your gluten-free journey. This lifestyle doesn't need to be an obstacle or a punishment — you simply need a shift in perspective and a wealth of top notch recipes that not only you can rely on, but that your friends will love too.

Coconut & Chia Fruit Stack Pot

SERVES 4

5 tbsp chia seeds

250ml / 1 cup almond milk

3 tbsp coconut cream

generous glug of maple syrup
or honey

130g / 3 cups coconut flakes

250g / 1¼ cups thick Greek
yoghurt

150g / 5¼oz fresh coconut
chunks

70g / 2½oz dried mango

1 ripe mango, peeled and
diced

Begin by combining the chia seeds, almond milk, coconut cream and maple syrup or honey in a bowl.

Cover and place in the fridge for at least 3–4 hours, or overnight.

When ready to serve, remove from the fridge and stir through half of the coconut flakes.

Add a spoonful of yoghurt to each serving dish, then layer up the chia pudding with more yoghurt.

Top each dish with the fresh coconut, remaining coconut flakes and both the dried and fresh mango.

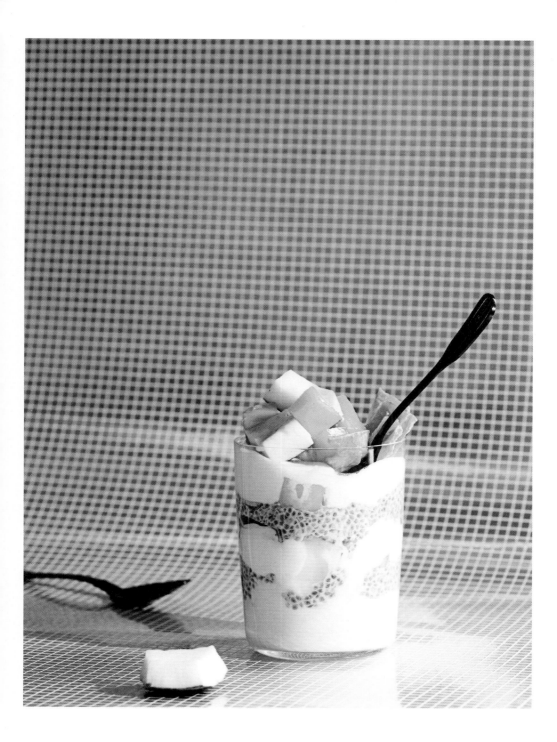

Quinoa & Cardamom Porridge / Honey Roasted Grapes

SERVES 4

125g / ⅔ cup cooked black or white quinoa (follow the cooking instructions on the packet for the quinoa, as these differ across varieties)

650ml / 2¾ cups almond milk (optional)

1 vanilla pod, seeds scraped out and reserved

4–6 drops of cardamom extract

3 tbsp chia seeds

120g / ½ cup extra-thick Greek yoghurt, plus extra to serve (optional)

TOPPING

1 large bunch of red grapes
generous drizzle of honey
squeeze of lemon juice

Preheat the oven to 190°C / 375°F/ gas mark 5.

Cut the bunch of grapes into four smaller bunches, one for each serving. Place on a baking tray (pan). Drizzle them with a little honey and a squeeze of lemon juice, and roast in the oven for around 15–20 minutes, or until the skins begin to blister a little.

In a saucepan, combine the cooked quinoa with 600ml / 2½ cups almond milk or water. Add in the vanilla pod and seeds, cardamom extract, chia seeds and the yoghurt.

Cook over a medium–low heat for 4–5 minutes, stirring until heated through. Add the remaining almond milk if it starts to become too thick.

Serve with an extra dollop of yoghurt, if you like, and the roasted grapes, plus a little extra honey to taste.

/ **Before cooking, you can 'activate' the quinoa. Place the grains in a bowl of chilled water, cover with parchment paper or clingfilm (plastic wrap), and refrigerate overnight. This isn't essential but makes the quinoa easier to digest.**

/ **Double the quantities to make enough porridge to last for the next couple of days. Allow to cool then refrigerate in a covered container. Reheat as required.**

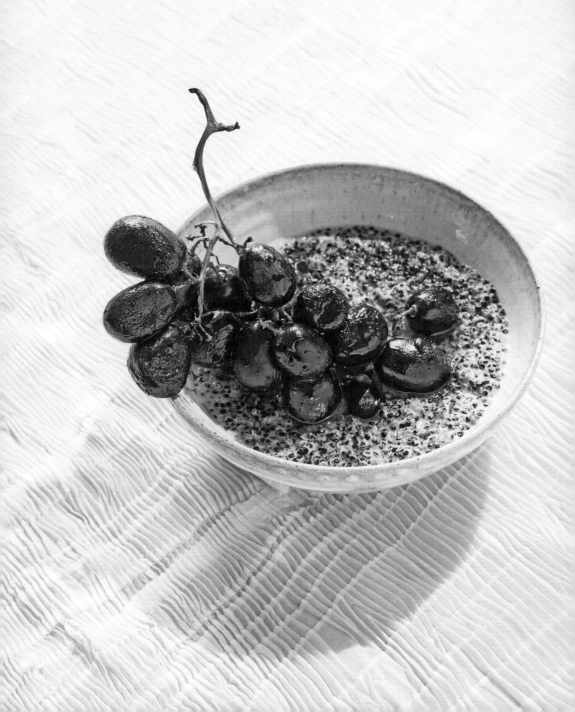

Green Pancakes

SERVES 2

FILLING

5 heaped tbsp ricotta

¼ freshly grated nutmeg

½ bunch of fresh parsley

bunch of fresh chives

100g / ⅔ cup peas, fresh or
  frozen (defrosted if frozen)

salt and freshly ground
  black pepper

PANCAKES

3 large eggs, beaten

3 handfuls of spinach

knob of butter

handful of fresh parsley,
  chopped

rapeseed (canola) oil, for
  frying

**/ Any fresh herbs will
work in these vibrant
pancakes, so use
whichever ones you
like or have to hand.**

Place the ricotta in a bowl with the grated nutmeg, a generous pinch of sea salt and plenty of black pepper, then mix together, taste for seasoning and adjust to your preference. Set to one side.

Place all of the pancake ingredients (apart from the oil) in a food processor with a generous pinch of sea salt and plenty of black pepper and blitz until combined into a smooth vibrant green liquid.

Heat a generous glug of oil in a large frying pan over a medium heat. Once hot, pour in one large ladleful (about half) of the green egg mixture and allow to almost cook through. The egg will no longer be completely runny but still not quite cooked.

Next spoon in half the ricotta filling onto one half of the pancake and add in half the parsley, chives and peas.

Fold the pancake over the filling and allow to cook for a further 30 seconds or so, just to heat the ricotta through a little. Carefully remove from the pan and keep warm while you cook the second pancake in the same way. Finish by sprinkling over a little extra seasoning.

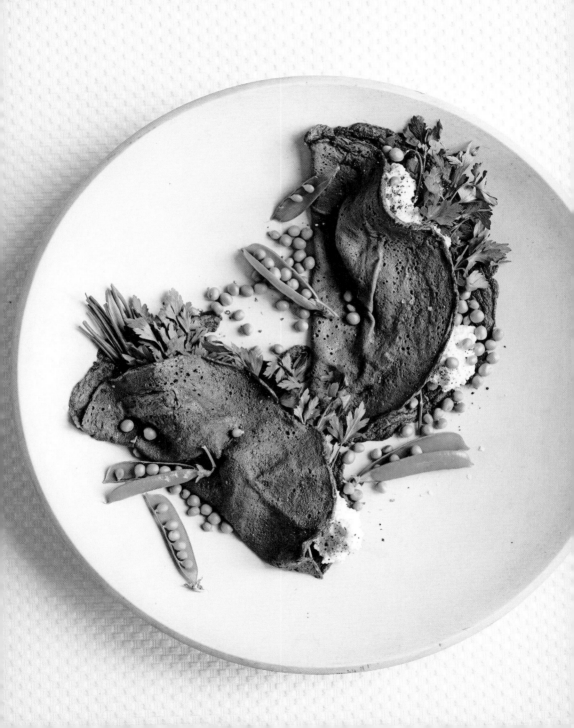

Know what to avoid...

/ Barley

/ Wheat

/ Bran

/ Spelt

/ Semolina

/ Malt (including vinegar)

/ Seitan

/ Rye

/ Egg noodles

/ Couscous

/ Beer / larger / ale / stout

/ Gravy granules

/ Pasta

/ Bread

/ Some ice cream

/ Most ready meals

Where's that gluten hiding?

Processed food / be cautious about any food that's been processed in any way, i.e. comes in a packet (you're always safe with fresh meat, fish, fruit and vegetables)

Thickeners / flours are often used to thicken sauces and soups

Breadcrumbs / be wary of anything with a crispy crumb

Stock / homemade stock should be fine, but shop-bought cubes usually contain gluten

Croutons / these nuggets are often omitted from menu descriptions; be sure to request 'no croutons' when ordering salads or soups

Fried food / deep fat fryers are often filled with tiny bits of batter or bread floating in the oil. So it's best to avoid anything dipped in fat when eating out

...but deny denial! Focus on the things you can enjoy*

All the vegetables

All the fruit

Beans

Pulses (including lentils)

Polenta

Potatoes

And, yes, quinoa

Cheese

All varieties of rice, including rice noodles and rice pasta

Meat

Fish

(Most) yoghurt

Did we say cheese?

Fruit juice

Cordials (not barley)

Fizzy soft drinks

Spirits

Cider

Wine / sherry

A lot of chocolate, including Wispa, Creme Egg, Flake, Crunchie, M&Ms and Toblerone**

* Always check the label as product manufacturing varies from country-to-country and from time-to-time.

** Please don't live on sweets and chocolate alone.

Buckwheat Chocolate Granola

SERVES 4–6

2 tbsp coconut oil

250g / 1½ cups buckwheat groats

150g / 1½ cups GF oats

150g / 2 cups desiccated (dried shredded) coconut

1 heaped tsp ground cinnamon

3–4 tbsp cocoa powder

5 drops of cardamom extract

1 tsp of vanilla bean paste

3 tbsp maple syrup

100g / 2 cups coconut flakes

2 tbsp pumpkin seeds

coconut yoghurt, Greek yoghurt or milk, to serve

Preheat the oven to 180°C / 360°F / gas mark 4. Line a large baking tray (pan) with parchment paper.

Melt the coconut oil in a saucepan over a medium–low heat until runny and set to one side.

Combine all the remaining ingredients in a bowl, reserving half the coconut flakes and the pumpkin seeds, then pour over the melted coconut oil, stirring so that everything is evenly coated.

Spread the mixture out onto the lined baking tray, in a single layer. Gently bake for 15 minutes before giving it a shake and baking for another 5–10 minutes, or until it begins to turn crisp.

On a separate non-stick baking tray (pan), or a tray lined with parchment paper, spread out the reserved coconut flakes and the pumpkin seeds and lightly toast in the oven for 4–5 minutes until the flakes begin to turn a little golden round the edges.

Combine the toasted coconut and pumpkin seeds with the cooked crunchy granola.

Serve with coconut yoghurt or thick Greek yoghurt, or simply add your favourite variety of milk.

Store any leftovers in an airtight container; it will keep for around a week.

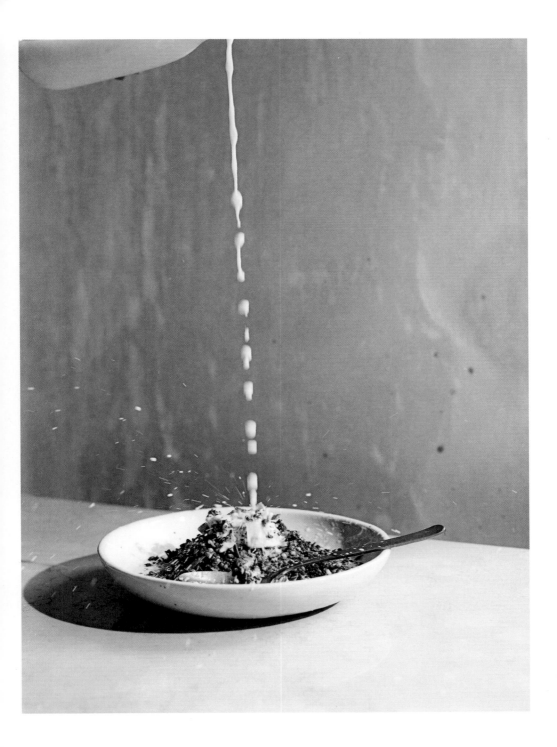

Fruit Pop Smoothies: Passion Fruit or Mango

MAKES 6–8 (depending on the size of the moulds)

4 tbsp honey, diluted with
   a splash of warm water
350ml / 1¾ cups extra-thick
   Greek yoghurt
juice of ½ orange
6–8 passion fruits or 2 very
   ripe mangos

Combine the honey, yoghurt and orange juice in a bowl.

Prepare the passion fruit or mango, whichever you are using. Scoop the flesh out of the passion fruit. Peel the mangos, roughly chop the flesh and blitz in a food processor until smooth.

Spoon the mixture into lolly or ice pop moulds, layering up the flavoured yoghurt and the fruit until all the mixture is used.

Take a knife and poke it in the bottom of each mould then drag it out, so that the layers combine just a little. Place the lids on, poke through the lolly sticks, and freeze for 2–3 hours.

/ These can be eaten as ice pops, ice lollies, or blitzed into a smoothie for a refreshing drink.

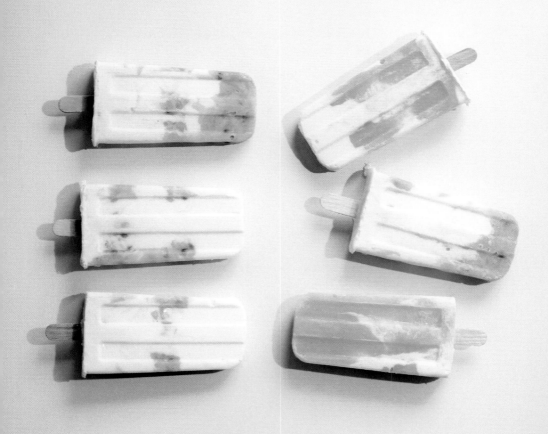

Coriander Baked Eggs / Yoghurt & Feta

SERVES 2

rapeseed (canola) oil

2 large handfuls of kale,
  roughly torn

bunch of fresh coriander
  (cilantro), stems trimmed,
  half roughly chopped, half
  left as is

6 tbsp extra-thick Greek
  yoghurt

150g / 5¼oz feta, crumbled

4 large organic free-range
  eggs

generous drizzle of Coriander
  (Cilantro) Oil (see page 81,
  optional)

salt and freshly ground
  black pepper

fresh or lightly toasted GF
  bread, to serve

Heat a generous glug of rapeseed (canola) oil in a large
frying pan or shallow casserole dish over a medium heat.
Add the kale to the pan and fry a little until wilted, then
add a generous sprinkle of salt and plenty of black pepper.

Next add the chopped half of the coriander (cilantro),
dot around the Greek yoghurt and scatter over half of the
crumbled feta.

Now crack in the eggs, one-by-one, leaving a gap between
each one. Continue to cook over a medium heat, covering
with a lid or foil for a minute or so to speed up the
cooking process.

Once then the eggs are cooked to your preference (around
2 minutes for poached but runny) drizzle over the
coriander oil, if using, and sprinkle with the whole sprigs
of coriander and the remaining feta.

Add a little extra seasoning and serve hot.

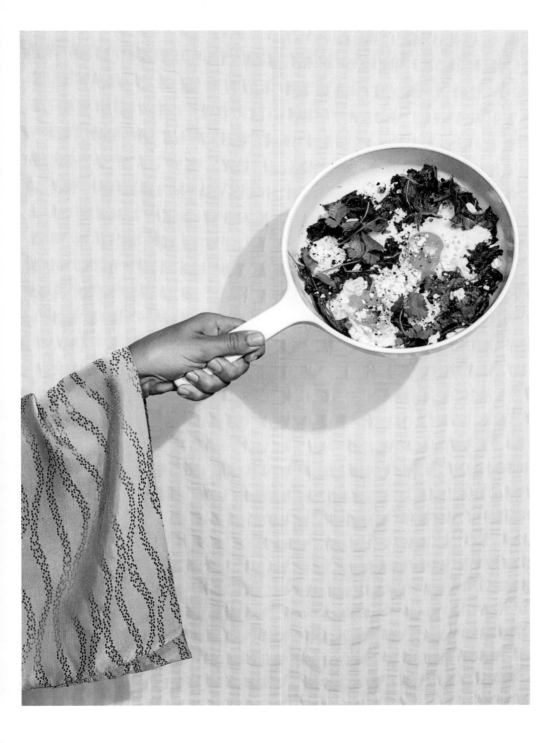

Buckwheat Crêpes / Scrambled Spiced Tofu / Refried Black Beans

//

MAKES 4–6

CRÊPES

100g / ¾ cup buckwheat flour

1 large egg

190ml / ¾ cup milk of
   your choice (non-dairy
   works too)

40g / 3 tbsp butter, melted

glug of rapeseed (canola)
   or olive oil

sea salt and freshly ground
   black pepper

REFRIED BEANS

generous glug of rapeseed
   (canola) or olive oil

½ onion, diced

2 cloves garlic, minced

2 x 400g / 14oz cans black
   beans, drained

1 tsp ground cumin

1 tsp smoked paprika

SCRAMBLED TOFU

generous glug of sesame oil

400g / 14oz GF silken tofu
   (beancurd), crumbled

½ tsp ground coriander

½ tsp ground cumin

generous sprinkle of sea salt
   flakes

GARNISH

1 lime, quartered

small bunch of fresh coriander
   (cilantro), ends trimmed

150ml / ⅔ cup sour cream

½ red onion, finely sliced

1 green chilli, finely sliced

First, combine all the crêpe ingredients, apart from the oil, in a large bowl, whisking until you have a smooth consistency. Season and place in the fridge.

Next make the refried beans. Heat a glug of oil over a medium heat and add the diced onion, cooking for several minutes until it softens and turns transparent. Add the garlic, cooking for another minute or so before adding the black beans, and spices. Season. >>>

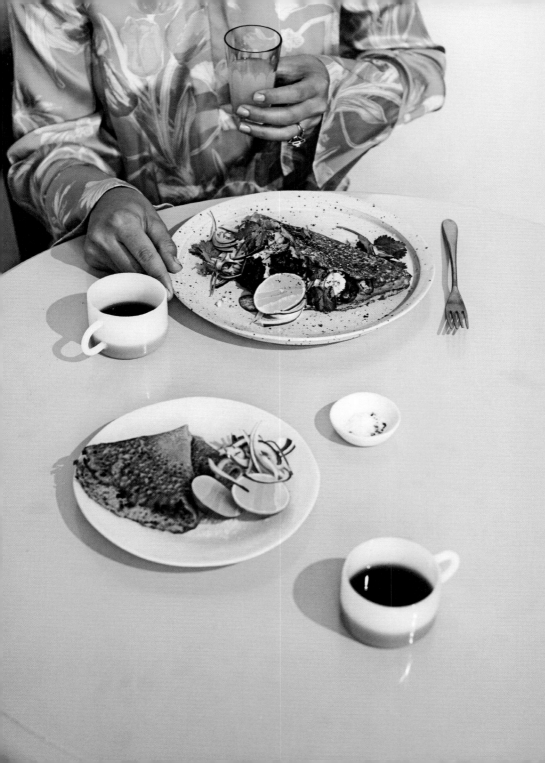

〰〰〰〰〰〰〰〰〰〰〰〰〰〰〰〰〰〰〰〰〰〰〰〰〰〰〰〰〰〰〰〰〰〰〰

>>> Mash the black beans with a potato masher or use the back of a spoon. Continue to cook over a medium–low heat for around 10 minutes to allow the flavours to come together. Keep warm until ready to serve.

For the scrambled tofu, in a separate pan, heat the sesame oil over a medium–high heat. Once hot, add in the crumbled tofu, followed by the spices and seasoning, and allow to cook for several minutes until it crisps up a little. Keep warm until ready to serve.

To make the crêpes, drizzle a little oil into a non-stick pan then wipe away the oil with kitchen paper to leave a lightly greased pan. Remove the crêpe batter from the fridge. Add a ladleful of the crêpe mixture to the pan and swirl it around so that you have a thin and even, round crêpe (you don't have to be fastidious about this, a roughly round crêpe will be fine).

Cook for 40–50 seconds then flip it over and cook the other side. Keep warm until ready to serve by wrapping in foil. Repeat with another ladle of crêpe batter until it is all used up.

Place the stack of cooked crêpes on the table with the beans, the scrambled tofu and the garnishes. Allow everyone to make up their own buckwheat crêpes – start with the refried beans, then add the scrambled tofu, followed by a dollop of sour cream and a selection of all the garnishes.

/ Not a tofu fan? You can also use regular scrambled eggs. Always add seasoning to eggs after cooking, rather than before, to avoid a watery consistency.

Embrace international flavours when eating in or out: good Indian food is often surprisingly gluten free (fresh curries, chickpea-flour bread, rice), while Mexican food is a saviour (corn tortilla wraps, rice, beans, cheese). In fact, a Mexican feast is a great thing to serve if you have people round for dinner (and is a great thing to suggest to a friend who feels terror at the thought of having you over).

Japanese-style Pancake

SERVES 1–2

several generous glugs of
    sesame oil
kernels from 2 sweetcorn
    cobs (ears of corn)
¼ head pointed spring greens
    or white cabbage, finely
    shredded on a mandolin
small bunch of fresh coriander
    (cilantro), leaves picked and
    roughly chopped
2 spring onions (scallions),
    finely sliced
generous sprinkle of sea salt
    flakes
½ tsp white pepper
½ green chilli, finely diced
3 large eggs, beaten
40g / ½ cup grated mature
    (sharp) Cheddar

HORSERADISH MAYONNAISE

3 tbsp good-quality
    mayonnaise
dash of yuzu or white wine
    vinegar
2–3 tsp grated fresh or
    creamed horseradish
sprinkle of sea salt flakes

To make the horseradish mayonnaise, simply combine all the ingredients in a bowl, adjusting the heat by adding more or less horseradish to your taste. Set aside.

Heat the sesame oil over a medium heat, add in the corn kernels and cook for a minute or so until the corn becomes vibrant yellow.

Add in the remaining ingredients, apart from the eggs and cheese, and fry for around 2 minutes.

Preheat the grill (broiler) to medium heat.

Next, combine half of the grated cheese with the beaten eggs, then pour the mixture over the greens and corn and allow to cook for 2–3 minutes over a medium heat.

Sprinkle the remaining cheese over the top and place under the grill for 2–3 minutes or until the cheese and edges start to crisp up.

Serve while warm, with the horseradish mayo drizzled over the top.

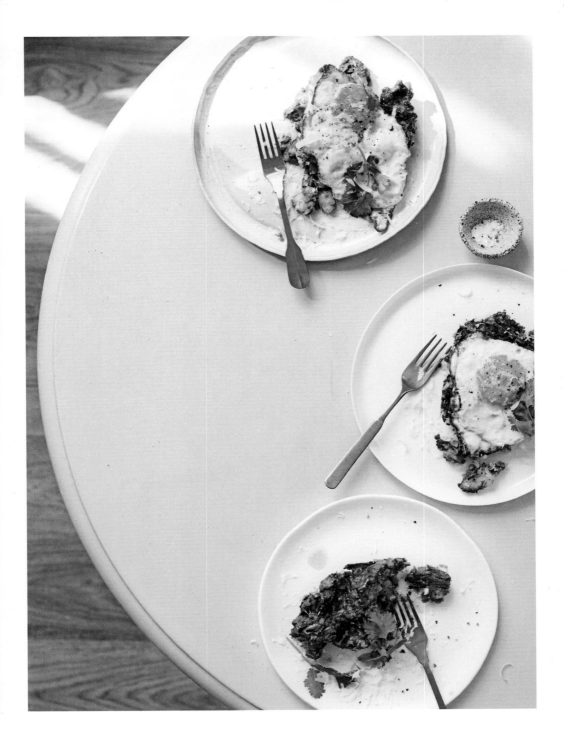

Banana Waffles
/ Salted Chocolate Sauce

SERVES 4

BANANA WAFFLES

425g / 3¼ cups GF
  wholemeal flour
1 tbsp baking powder
generous sprinkle of sea salt
280ml / 1¼ cups coconut
  milk
2 overripe bananas;
  1 mashed, 1 chopped into
  small chunks
½ tsp vanilla extract or ¼ tsp
  vanilla bean paste
2 eggs
125ml / ½ cup rapeseed
  (canola) oil
butter or coconut oil, for
  greasing

TOPPING

1 punnet of strawberries,
  about 350g / 12oz, hulled
  and quartered

3 tbsp sugar or honey
  (optional)
squeeze of lemon juice
  (optional)

SALTED CHOCOLATE SAUCE

200g / 7oz good-quality dark
  chocolate
175ml / ¾ cup double
  (heavy) cream
50ml / 3½ tbsp full-fat milk
½ tsp vanilla bean paste
generous sprinkle of sea
  salt flakes
1 tbsp butter (optional)

TO SERVE

6–8 fresh strawberries
icing (confectioners') sugar,
  to dust (optional)

Preheat the oven to 150°C / 300°F / gas mark 2.

Whisk together all the waffle ingredients, apart from the
butter or oil for greasing and the banana, in a large bowl
until you have a smooth mixture, then refrigerate until
ready to use.

To make a quick strawberry compote, add all the topping
ingredients to a saucepan, cover and cook for 3–4 minutes
or until it becomes syrupy. >>>

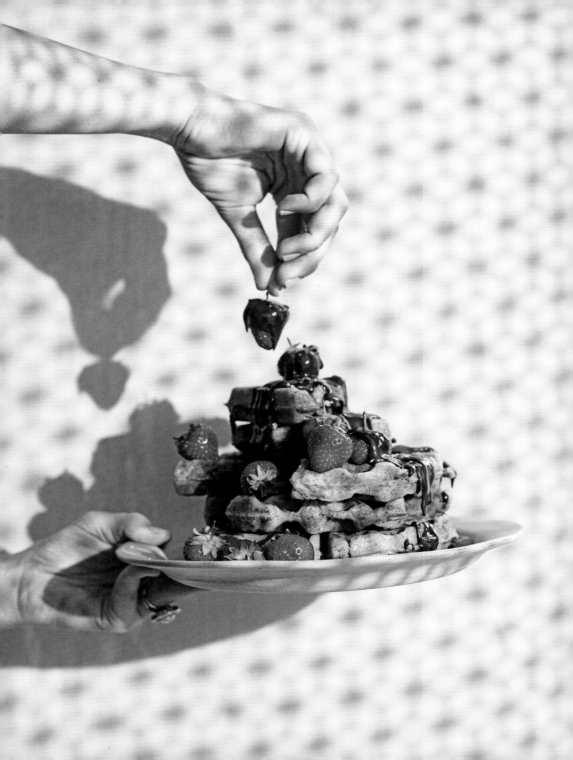

>>> Alternatively, reserve the fresh strawberries and simply use them to top the waffles when serving.

For the salted chocolate sauce, combine everything except the butter in a saucepan and warm over a low–medium heat, stirring to ensure there are no lumps. For extra glossiness, add the tablespoon of butter to the sauce. Check the flavour and add more salt depending on how prominent you want the saltiness to be. Keep warm.

Heat the waffle iron and coat with either melted butter or coconut oil. Add several pieces of the chopped banana to the iron, then pour over a small ladleful of the waffle mixture. Close the irons, cooking until golden and crisp. Once cooked, keep warm in the oven while you cook the remaining waffle batter in the same way.

To serve, stack the waffles, layering them up with the compote or fresh strawberries. Pour over the chocolate sauce and dust with icing (confectioners') sugar, if using.

Brunch is one of life's simple joys — don't miss out by believing toast is the be-all. Think bigger: kedgeree topped with a steaming egg; halloumi with a side of grilled toms, spinach and beans; or a loaded corn tortilla. All yum!

Egg Hoppers
/ Sri Lankan Fried Chicken

||||||||||||||||||||||||||||||||||||||

SERVES 4

EGG HOPPERS

7g / ¼oz dried yeast

1 tbsp golden caster
  (superfine) sugar

250g / 2 cups rice flour

500ml / 2¼ cups coconut
  milk

glug of olive oil, for frying

4 eggs

sea salt flakes and white
  pepper

FRIED CHICKEN

4–6 chicken thighs

100g / ¾ cup chickpea
  (gram) flour

2 tbsp cornflour (cornstarch)

2 tbsp desiccated (dried
  shredded) coconut

1 tsp smoked paprika

½ tsp white pepper

sprinkle of sea salt flakes

zest of 1 lime

2 free-range eggs, beaten

500ml / 2¼ cups vegetable
  oil, for frying

GARNISH

1 lime, quartered

several sprigs of fresh
  coriander (cilantro)

First make the hoppers. Combine 120ml / ½ cup room-temperature water with the yeast and sugar. Leave for around 8–10 minutes or until it begins to foam.

Place the rice flour in a bowl with the coconut milk, then add the water and yeast mixture. Stir until combined, season with a sprinkle of sea salt flakes plus a dash of white pepper, and leave overnight in the fridge.

To cook the hoppers, remove the batter from the fridge, bring to room temperature and whisk to remove any lumps. Add a good glug of water if the consistency is too thick – it should be a runny batter.

Preheat the oven to 150°C / 300°F / gas mark 2.

Heat a round non-stick, high-sided wok-style pan over a medium heat. Brush over a little oil, covering the entire pan, then wipe off with kitchen paper.

Add a small ladle of the batter and immediately swirl it round the pan to create the high edges in the shape of a bowl. Cook for around a minute then crack an egg into the centre of the bottom of the hopper. Cook for a further 2–3 minutes over a medium heat, until the egg is cooked and the edges begin to turn a little golden.

Remove from the pan and repeat until you have four egg hoppers. Place in the oven to keep warm.

For the fried chicken, cut away some of the meat on the chicken thighs, so you still have the bone with some meat on, but also a second separate piece of meat. >>>

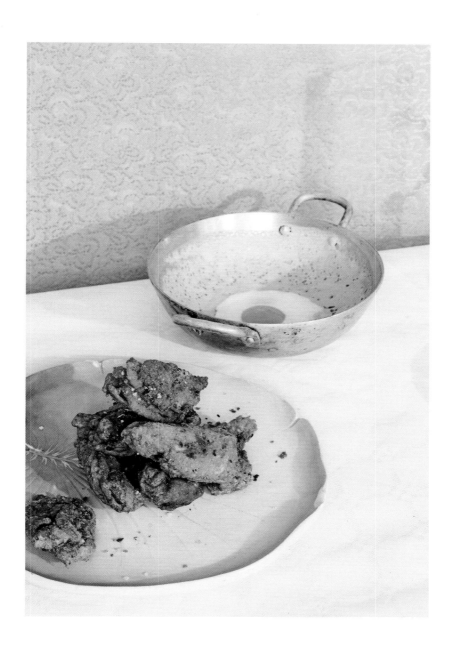

>>> Combine the flours, coconut, paprika, pepper, salt and lime zest in a small bowl.

Dunk each piece of chicken into the beaten egg, then thoroughly pat the dry coating all over the pieces of chicken.

Set the chicken pieces to one side and, in a large saucepan, heat the vegetable oil to 180°C / 360°F. In batches, so you don't overload your pan, cook the chicken pieces until crispy and the chicken is cooked through – this should take around 4–5 minutes depending on how large your chicken thighs are. Remember to allow the oil to come back up to temperature ahead of cooking each batch of chicken. Once cooked drain the oil off on kitchen paper.

Serve the fried chicken with the egg hoppers, lime wedges and fresh coriander (cilantro).

There's always an app...

Whichever packet of processed food you're peering at intensely, and whatever menu you're trying to navigate, believe that someone has been there before you. To save your eyes from scanning the small print, draw on the experience of others and download a credible app. In the UK, Coeliac UK offers the Gluten Free Food Checker and the Gluten Free On the Move apps to help you make fuss-free decisions.

Tuna Sambal Broth / Vermicelli Noodles

SERVES 4

1l / 4¼ cups good-quality fish
  stock
3 stalks lemongrass, ends
  trimmed and bashed
5cm / 2in piece of fresh root
  ginger, peeled and finely
  grated
3–4 tbsp sambal oelek
  (minced red chillies),
  to taste
350g / 12oz rice vermicelli
  noodles
dash of tamari or fish
  sauce (optional)
350–450g / 12–16oz fresh
  sushi-grade tuna, roughly
  cut into 4 steaks
sesame oil, to drizzle
large bunch of fresh Thai basil
small bunch of fresh mint,
  leaves picked
2 limes, quartered

Begin by bringing the fish stock to the boil, then add the lemongrass and ginger and cook for around 10 minutes. Add in the sambal oelek, a spoonful at a time and taste the broth to ensure it's not too spicy.

Next cook your vermicelli noodles as per the packet instructions and set to one side.

When you're ready to serve, simply make sure the broth is boiling (and that you're happy with the flavour – add a little tamari or fish sauce for more saltiness if needed). Add the fillets of tuna to the broth and allow to poach for a minute.

Divide the noodles across four serving bowls, then pour over the broth. Arrange the fresh tuna on top of the noodles, so it's submerged in the broth.

Drizzle with sesame oil and scatter over a generous amount of Thai basil and fresh mint. Finish with a squeeze of fresh lime and serve.

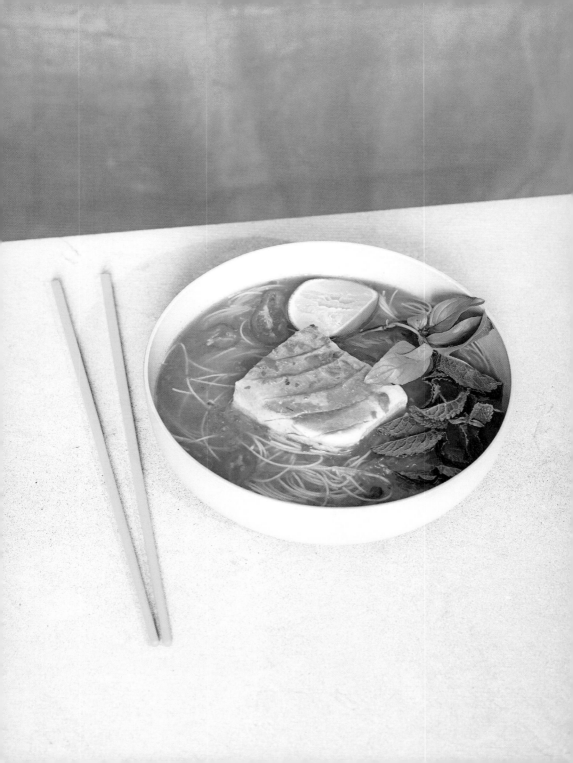

Roasted Chicken / Kale Caesar Salad

////////////////////////////////

SERVES 4–6

2 onions, quartered

small bunch of fresh thyme

1 large free-range corn fed
   chicken, around 1.5–1.8kg
   (3lb 5oz–4lb)

glug of olive oil

220g / 8oz kale, stalks
   removed and leaves roughly
   chopped or torn

6–12 good-quality anchovies
   in oil, to taste

40g / ½ cup finely grated
   Parmesan (optional if you
   prefer a dairy-free salad)

Corn Chips with Thyme Salt
   (see page 88)

zest and juice of ½ lemon

salt and freshly ground
   black pepper

DRESSING

1 tsp tahini (sesame paste)

2 tbsp sweet white miso paste

100ml / generous ⅓ cup
   olive oil

freshly ground black pepper

Preheat the oven to 200°C / 400°F / gas mark 6.

Place the quartered onions and thyme in a large roasting pan. Season the chicken and place it on top of the onions in the tray, upside down.

Roast according to the instructions on the packaging. Depending on the weight, this could be anything from 50 minutes to 1 hour 20 minutes.

Three-quarters of the way into its cooking time, turn the chicken so that it is breast side up, to crisp up the skin. Pierce the flesh of the thickest part of the thigh with a skewer – when it is cooked, the juices will run clear. Remove from the oven and allow to rest for at least 15 minutes.

Place the kale in a large bowl. Combine the dressing ingredients. Taste and adjust the seasoning to your preference, then pour the dressing over the kale, thoroughly coating it and massaging it into the kale. Place in the fridge for 10–15 minutes to allow the kale to soften a little.

When ready to serve, pull the meat off the chicken, shredding it into bite-sized portions, and combine with the kale. Add the anchovies, Parmesan shavings, corn chips, lemon zest and a squeeze of lemon juice. Season to taste, being careful to not overdo the salt as the anchovies will add a lot of saltiness to this dish.

Alternatively, serve the chicken whole with the kale on the side and let everyone tuck in.

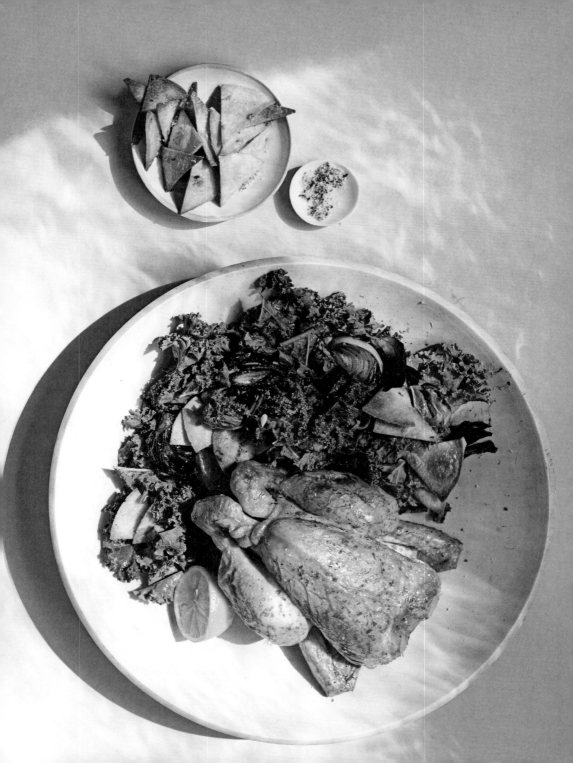

Roasted Garlic, Ricotta & Asparagus Tarts

SERVES 4

1 garlic bulb

250g / 1 cup ricotta

150g / ¾ cup mascarpone

2 eggs

200g / 7oz baby asparagus,
  ends trimmed or peeled

drizzle of olive oil

salt and freshly ground
  black pepper

SHORT CRUST PASTRY
(optional, readymade can also
  be used)

240g / 1¾ cups GF plain
  (all-purpose) flour, sieved,
  plus extra for dusting

sprinkle of salt

110g / ½ cup chilled unsalted
  butter, cubed

1 tsp Dijon mustard

1 egg, beaten, plus 1 yolk
  for glazing

4 sprigs of fresh thyme, leaves
  removed from stalks

3–4 tbsp ice-cold water

If making homemade pastry, start by using a stand mixer with the K beater to mix the flour with the salt, then add in the butter, combining on a low speed until you have a rough crumb.

Next add the Dijon mustard and the egg. When the pastry starts to come together add in the thyme leaves and ice-cold water, a tablespoon at a time, adding just enough of the water so that the pastry forms a smooth ball. If you add too much you can add a little extra flour to bring it back to the right texture.

Remove the dough from the food processor, roll it out a little then wrap in cling film (plastic wrap) or parchment paper and allow to rest in the fridge for 30 minutes.

Preheat the oven to 180°C / 360°F / gas mark 4.

Wrap the bulb of garlic in foil and place in the oven for around 20–25 minutes until the cloves are soft.

Once the pastry is ready, use it to line four small (5–6cm/ 2–2½in) tart cases or one large (24–26cm/9½–10½in) one.

Roll out the pastry on a floured surface to around 5mm / ¼in thick. Line your tart tin or tins, leaving about 1cm / ½in extra pastry overhanging the edge.

Prick the base of the pastry case(s) several times with a fork. Fill the bottom of the tart tin(s) with baking beans and blind bake your pastry for 15–20 minutes. >>>

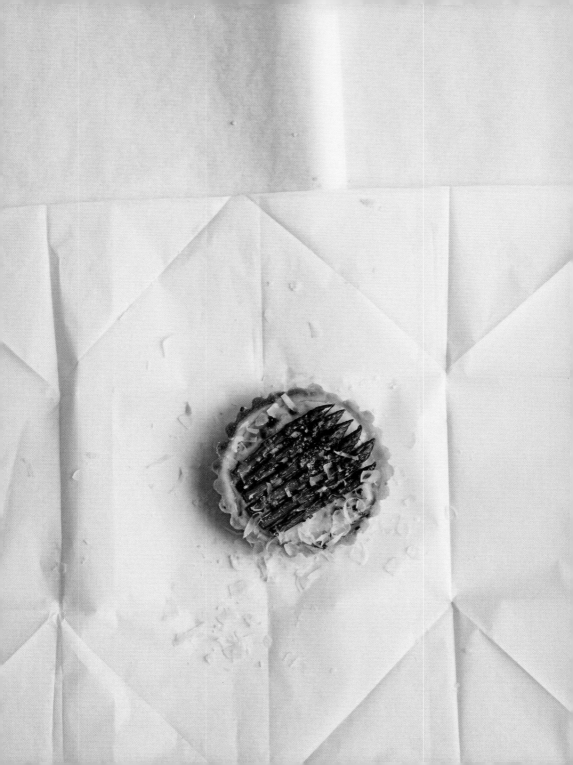

>>> Place the egg yolk in a small bowl and whisk.

Remove the pastry case from the oven, take out the beans and trim the excess pastry. Then brush the whisked egg yolk over the pastry and return to the oven and bake for another 5 minutes.

For the filling, simply combine the roasted garlic (squeezing the flesh out of the skins) with the ricotta, mascarpone, eggs and seasoning and pour into the pastry tart case(s).

Lay the baby asparagus on top, add a drizzle of oil and place back in the oven for around 12–15 minutes until the ricotta has set. Serve warm or chilled.

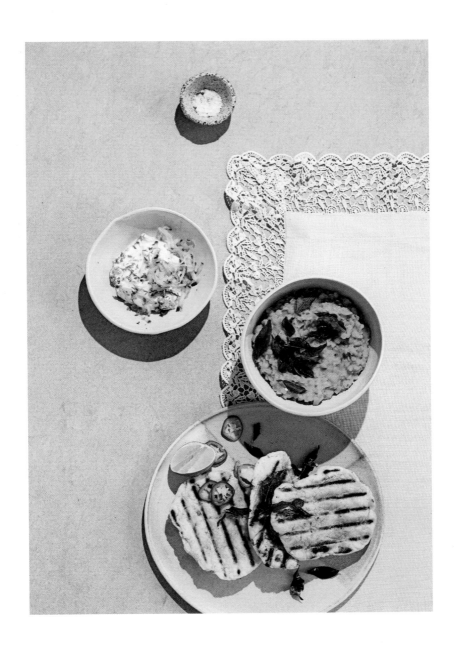

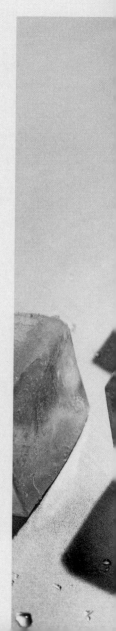

>>> Next add the spices, followed by the lentils. Stir thoroughly then add the coconut milk and 200ml / scant 1 cup water. Simmer over a medium–low heat for around 15–20 minutes.

For the flatbreads, combine the flour, coriander (cilantro), cumin, seasoning and lemon zest. Add the yoghurt and 80ml / ⅓ cup water, combining until you have a dough.

Divide into 6 pieces, then roll out into around 5mm / ¼in thick medium-sized rounds.

Sprinkle with a little extra gluten-free flour to help prevent any sticking.

Heat a griddle pan until almost smoking then place the flatbreads on the griddle for around 30–40 seconds on each side or until they puff up. You can also place under the grill (broiler), cooking for around 3–4 minutes or until golden on each side.

Combine all of the raita ingredients in a small bowl.

For the crispy curry leaves, heat the coconut or rapeseed (canola) oil, then once hot, add in the leaves and fry for about 20–30 seconds until they are dark in colour.

Remove the leaves from the oil and drain on kitchen paper. Sprinkle the crispy curry leaves over the top of the daal and the flatbreads. Add the chilli and lime to the flatbreads, and serve with the daal.

Ice, ice, baby

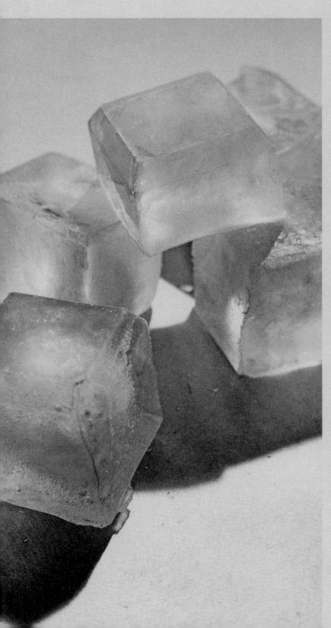

Push that bag of peas to one side and make use of all of that cavernous space in your freezer. On days when there is 'nothing in', when people are dropping by last minute, or when you're just feeling super lazy, you'll be so thankful you made extra curry (see page 122), and thought to freeze those extra flatbreads (see page 96). Fill it, use it, learn to love it.

Parmesan Waffles
/ Confit Tomatoes & Burrata

SERVES 4

knob of butter or olive oil,
  to grease the waffle irons
200g / 1½ cups GF
  wholegrain flour
2 tsp GF baking powder
several turns of freshly
  ground black pepper
1 egg
180ml / ¾ cup milk or milk
  alternative
60ml / ¼ cup olive or
  rapeseed (canola) oil
2 spring onions (scallions),
  finely sliced
150g / 2 cups finely
  grated Parmesan

TO SERVE

1 ball of burrata, quartered
generous dollop of Confit
  tomatoes (see page 72)
several sprigs of fresh thyme,
  leaves picked from the stem
drizzle of maple syrup

Begin by measuring out the ingredients for the waffles.
Allow the waffle irons to heat up. Brush generously with
butter or oil.

Combine the flour, baking powder and pepper in a large
bowl. In another bowl combine the egg, milk and oil, then
gradually add the wet ingredients to the dry.

Stir thoroughly, then fold in the spring onions (scallions)
and Parmesan and spoon half of the mixture into the
waffle iron.

Cook until golden and crisp. You can keep the waffles
warm in the oven (preheated to 150°C / 300°F / gas
mark 2), while you make up your second batch.

Serve the waffles topped with the burrata and 1–2 generous
spoonfuls of confit tomatoes. Scatter over the thyme leaves
and finish with a little drizzle of maple syrup and extra
black pepper.

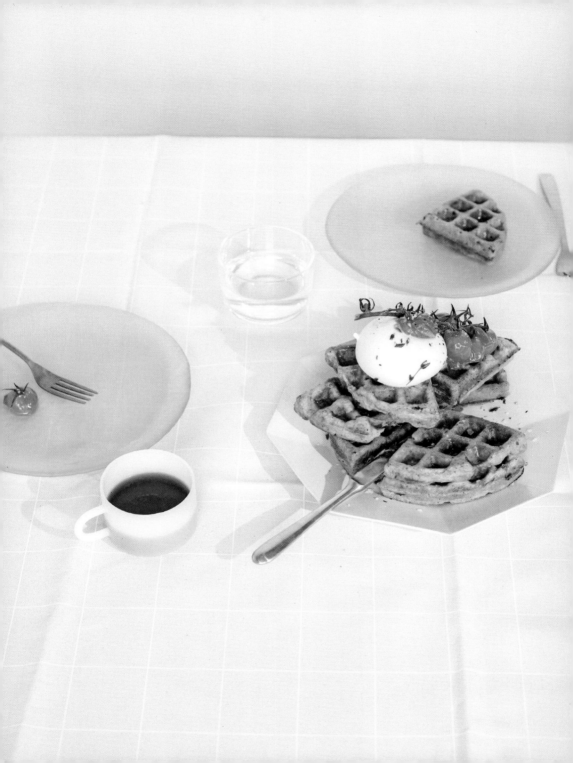

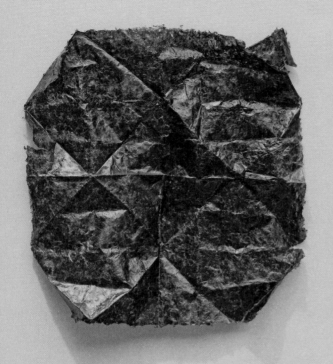

Sushi is
an ideal GF dish when made right. But beware of the pre-packaged stuff as, alas, shop-bought sushi is often full of hidden gluten.

Feeling crabby / Crab substitute is a favourite in budget sushi. Known as 'surimi', this paste is made by grinding down white fish meat, often with the addition of starch, until it resembles crab meat. Best just to avoid.

Less saucy / Sadly soy sauce is a no-go. Don't be caught out by fish that has been marinated in soy sauce and other sauces containing it, like teriyaki. Rice vinegar and wasabi may also contain traces of gluten, so be sure to check the label. You should be safe with tamarind sauce.

Batter chatter / Beware of tempura as the batter used is commonly made from wheat flour.

Sushi is super easy to make – learn to magic up some fancy-looking cones on page 50, then make yourself an easy packed lunch or a 'wow' dinner for friends.

If you're going out, obviously let the wait staff know about your allergies (make sure you impress how serious they are), then stick to the fresh sashimi. You can always whip out your own gluten-free soy sauce – don't feel embarrassed, embrace your lifestyle, live GF and proud, and snap your chop sticks together with sass!

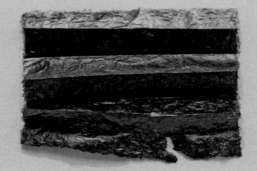

Black Rice Sushi Cones / Melted Camembert & Avocado

SERVES 4

220g / 1¼ cups black glutinous rice (it's glutinous and sticky, but still GF)
60ml / ¼ cup rice vinegar
1 tsp caster (superfine) sugar
sprinkle of sea salt flakes
4 sheets of nori, each halved to make two rectangles about 4 x 7cm (1½ x 2¾in)

FILLING

½ Camembert
1–2 tsp wasabi
1 ripe avocado, halved and cut into long strips
1 spring onion (scallion), finely sliced in half then lengthways into strips
small bunch of fresh coriander (cilantro), left as sprigs, ends trimmed

Preheat the oven to 170°C / 320°F/ gas mark 3.

First, cook the black rice as per the pack instructions (which may vary by brand). Once cooked (and liquid free, drain if necessary), add in the rice vinegar, sugar and a sprinkle of salt, thoroughly combine and transfer to a tray. Spread out and allow to cool.

Bake the Camembert. Place it in the preheated oven on a baking tray (pan) for 6–8 minutes or until runny. Meanwhile, prepare all the other filling ingredients and have them set out in front of you.

Spoon the cooled rice onto the halved nori sheets, spreading it just across half of the rectangle so you have a neat square of rice. Brush on a small amount of wasabi.

Place the avocado and spring onion (scallion) strips and the coriander (cilantro) on top of the rice, diagonally onto the square, with the bottom of the strips starting from the bottom right corner.

Once you've layered up your ingredients, drizzle over a little melted Camembert then roll each sheet into a cone. Use a little water to stick the end of the nori to round the cone shape. Drizzle over a little extra Camembert and serve.

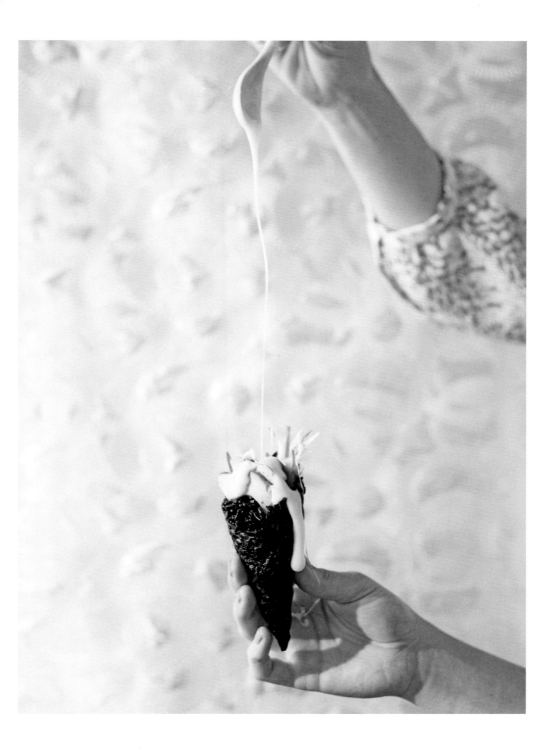

Pickled Rhubarb & Tuna Tostadas

SERVES 4

16 rice paper rounds

sesame oil, for frying

250–300g / 9–10½oz sushi
grade tuna, cubed

1 spring onion (scallion),
finely sliced

1 chilli, finely sliced

small bunch of fresh coriander
(cilantro), leaves picked

Coriander Oil (see page 81,
optional), to serve

PICKLED RHUBARB

125ml / ½ cup apple cider
vinegar

100g / ½ cup caster
(superfine) sugar

1 tsp black peppercorns

3 bird's eye chillies, pricked

1 bay leaf

200g / 7oz rhubarb, cut into
3¼–4cm / 1–1½in lengths

DRIZZLE

4 tbsp sesame oil

2 tbsp GF soy sauce

1 tbsp mirin

Place all the ingredients for the pickled rhubarb, except
the rhubarb, in a pan, add 125ml / ½ cup water, and bring
almost to the boil. Transfer to a sterilized jar and add the
chopped rhubarb. Allow to cool, then chill in the fridge
for 3–4 hours or ideally overnight.

For the tostadas, dip a rice paper round in warm water to
hydrate, fold it in half and then half again. Repeat to fold
all the rice paper.

Heat a generous glug of sesame oil in a large frying pan,
and once hot, fry each of the rice papers on both sides –
they should only take 20 seconds or so to blister up and
turn golden. You can do as many as you can fit in your
frying pan without them overlapping. Drain on kitchen
paper until ready to serve.

Combine the sesame oil, soy sauce and mirin to make
a sauce for drizzling.

Place the tuna, spring onion (scallion), chilli and
coriander (cilantro) on a platter with the rice papers,
for everyone to help themselves, or portion up on
individual plates.

Serve with the pickled rhubarb, the drizzle and some
coriander oil, if using.

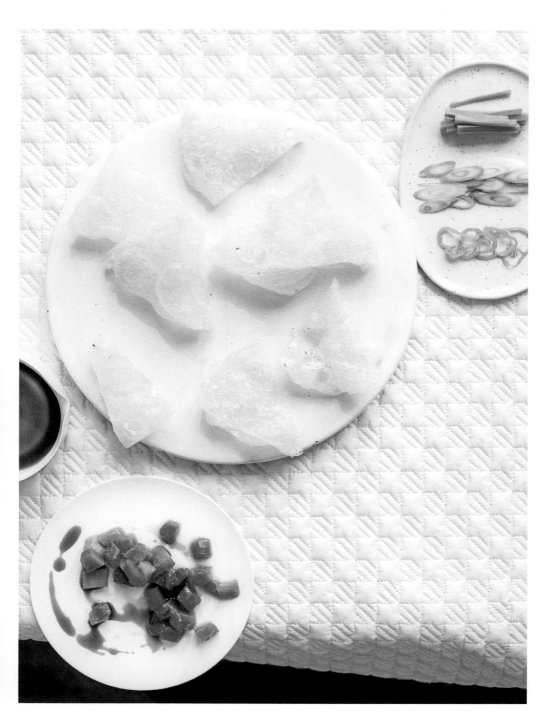

Poached Salmon Parcels / Ginger & Chicken Broth

SERVES 4

1 litre / 4¼ cups good-quality chicken broth

5cm / 2in piece of fresh root ginger, peeled and cut into matchsticks

2 stalks lemongrass, ends trimmed, halved and bashed

small bunch of fresh Thai basil

good dash of fish sauce

1 green chilli, finely sliced

sesame oil, to drizzle

SALMON PARCELS

350g / 12oz Chinese greens or morning glory

4 sustainable, responsibly sourced salmon fillets, around 180–200g / 6¼–7oz each

several glugs of tamari sauce

10cm / 4in piece of fresh root ginger, peeled and finely grated

2 cloves garlic, grated

½ bunch fresh Thai basil

Preheat the oven to 180°C / 360°F / gas mark 4.

Make the salmon parcels. Prepare four large, double-layered sheets of either parchment paper or foil, around 40 x 40cm (16 x 16in).

Place a layer of greens in each, then sit the salmon fillets on top. Add a glug of tamari sauce to each one, then add the ginger, garlic and Thai basil. Wrap up each parcel so it's airtight.

Place the salmon parcels in the oven on a baking tray (pan). Cook for around 12–15 minutes.

Meanwhile, put the chicken broth in a pan with the ginger, lemongrass, half the Thai basil and a dash of fish sauce, to taste.

Cook over a medium heat for 10–15 minutes then pour the broth into four serving bowls, and add the contents of one salmon parcel to each bowl.

Scatter with the remaining Thai basil and the green chilli, and add a drizzle of sesame oil.

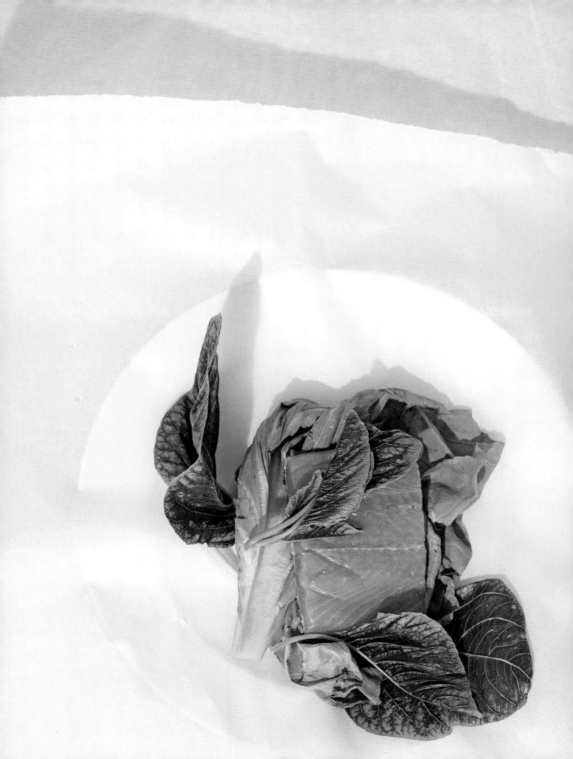

Matcha & Coconut Popcorn

SERVES 4–6

75g / 1¼ cups coconut flakes
50g / ¾ cup desiccated
  (dried shredded) coconut
75g / 2½oz plain popcorn
1 tsp matcha powder
50g / 2 cups puffed rice cereal
50ml / 3½ tbsp maple syrup

Preheat oven to 170°C / 320°F/ gas mark 3. Line a large baking tray (pan) with parchment paper.

Combine all the dry ingredients in a large bowl, then add the maple syrup and stir until everything is evenly coated. Transfer to the lined baking tray and bake for around 15–20 minutes, until the popcorn is just beginning to turn golden.

Remove from the oven and allow to cool before eating.

Store in an airtight container, where it will keep for about a week.

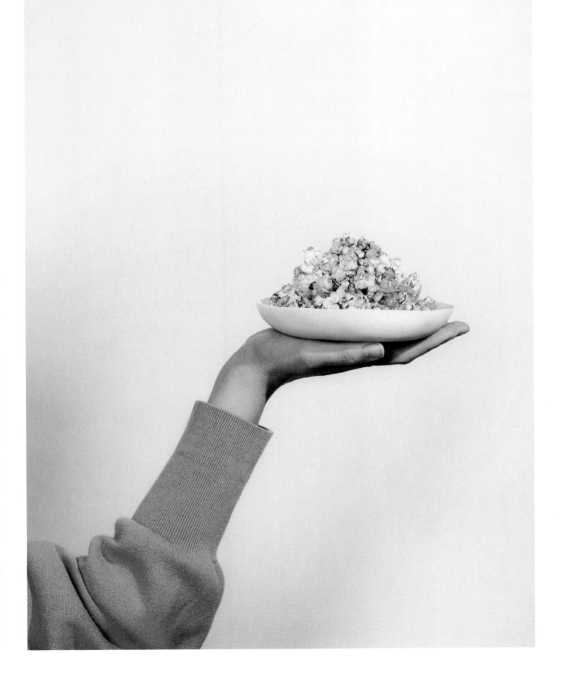

Pistachio, Matcha, Almond & Date Balls

\\

MAKES 8–12 BALLS

30g / ½ cup desiccated
   (dried shredded) coconut
2 tbsp matcha powder
120g / 1¼ cups ground
   almonds
260g / 1⅔ cups pistachios,
   shelled
6 Medjool dates, pitted

Place the desiccated coconut in a small bowl, add
1 tablespoon of the ground almonds and 1 teaspoon
of the matcha powder, and thoroughly combine.

In a food processor, blitz together the remaining matcha
powder and ground almonds with the pistachios and dates
until the mixture comes together to a thick paste, but is
not too wet. You can wet the balls with a little water before
rolling in the mixture for extra tackiness.

Roll the mixture into small balls (a little smaller than
a golf ball) with your hands. Finish by rolling each ball
through the coconut mixture.

Store in an airtight container. They should keep for
around a week or so.

Balls are pictured on page 60.

Puffed Rice, Peanut Butter & Dried Banana Nut Clusters

\\

MAKES 6–8

250g / 10 cups GF puffed rice cereal

70g / 1 cup dried banana, roughly chopped

60g / ½ cup cashews, roughly chopped

1 very ripe banana, mashed

3 tbsp coconut oil

80ml / 5½ tbsp maple syrup

4 tbsp peanut butter (smooth or crunchy)

Preheat the oven to 170°C / 320°F/ gas mark 3. Line a large baking tray (pan) with parchment paper or use a non-stick baking tray.

In a large bowl, combine the puffed rice cereal, dried banana and cashews. Stir through the mashed banana and coconut oil.

In a small bowl, mix together the maple syrup and peanut butter, adding a small dash of boiling water if needed, to make it into a looser paste.

Now stir the paste through the combined ingredients, evenly coating everything. Transfer the mixture to the baking tray, pressing evenly into the edges of the tray.

Bake for 12–15 minutes, or until it begins to turn golden and sets. Allow to cool a little, then slice or break into clusters of whatever size you prefer.

Store in an airtight container. They will keep for around 3–4 days.

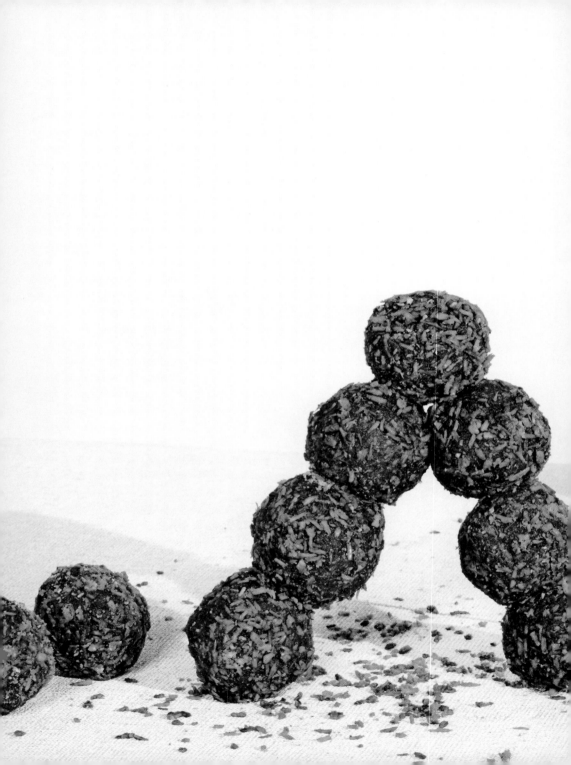

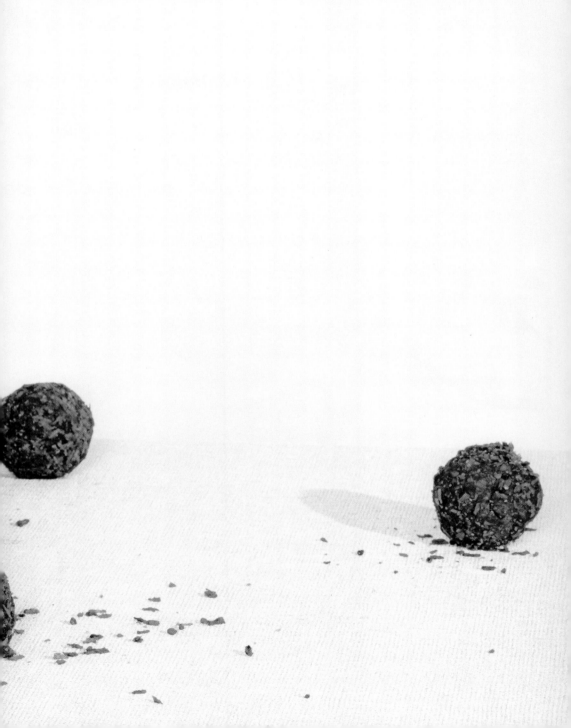

Nut, Seed & Cranberry Loaf / Almond Butter

SERVES 4–6

100g / ¾ cup pumpkin seeds

100g / ¾ cup cashews

100g / ¾ cup almonds

100g / ¾ cup hazelnuts

100g / ¾ cup pistachios, shelled

100g / ¾ cup dried cranberries

5 eggs, beaten

100ml / generous ⅓ cup extra virgin olive oil

1 large pinch sea salt flakes

TOPPING

130g / ½ cup almond butter

3 bananas, sliced

1 tbsp chia seeds or other mixed seeds

Preheat the oven to 160°C / 325°F / gas mark 2–3. Grease a 25cm (10in) loaf tin (pan) with a little oil.

Mix all the loaf ingredients together in a bowl. Transfer to the greased loaf tin and bake for 55 minutes.

Let cool slightly in the tin, then transfer to a cooling rack. Serve while warm or allow to cool completely.

To serve, slice the loaf, then add the toppings. Add a layer of almond butter, followed by fresh sliced ripe banana and a small sprinkle of chia seeds or mixed seeds.

Store the bread (unsliced) in an airtight container and keep refrigerated. It will last for up to a week.

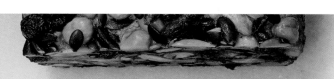

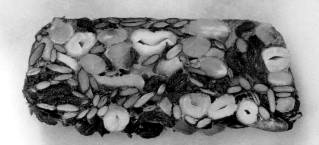

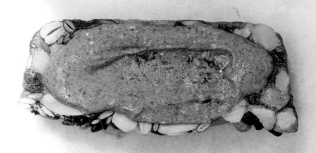

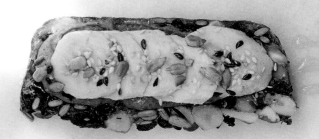

Wholemeal Soda Bread

MAKES 1 LOAF

360g / 2¾ cups GF
  wholemeal flour, plus
  extra for dusting
90g / 1 cup GF oats
8g / 1½ tsp sea salt flakes,
  ground
20g / 1½ tbsp GF bicarbonate
  of soda (baking soda)
4 egg yolks
300ml / 1¼ cups buttermilk
  or plain yoghurt (or full-fat
  milk mixed with 1 tbsp
  lemon juice)
milk, for glazing

Preheat the oven to 180°C / 360°F / gas mark 4.

Combine all the dry ingredients in a large bowl: flour, oats, salt and bicarbonate of soda (baking soda). Make a well in the middle and add in 50ml / 3½ tbsp water, the egg yolks, and the buttermilk, yoghurt or milk. Combine until you have a smooth, dough-like consistency.

Roll the dough into a round or oval shape and score the top with your choice of design. Crosshatch works well. Brush over a splash of milk with a pastry brush.

Prepare a heavy-based dish – ideally a casserole pot around 22cm / 8½in – by lightly brushing with water then sprinkling over a layer of GF flour. Place the bread dough in the dish. The flour will help it to not stick.

To create steam and give the bread a good layer of crunch to its crust, place a heatproof bowl in the bottom of the oven and add a good glug of water to it. Top the water up halfway through cooking.

Sprinkle a little extra flour on top of the dough and place in the oven for around 8–10 minutes.

After this time, reduce the heat to 160°C / 325°F / gas mark 2–3 and continue to bake for a further 15 minutes, or until you have a golden loaf.

Remove the loaf from the dish and allow to cool on a wire rack.

Olive & Oregano Plait Loaf

MAKES 1 LOAF

500g / 3¾ cups GF
  wholemeal flour

1 tsp salt

7g / ¼oz dried yeast

2 tbsp golden caster
  (superfine) sugar

75g / ⅓ cup butter, melted

350ml / 1½ cups full-fat milk,
  plus extra for glazing

2 eggs, beaten

1 tsp apple cider vinegar

150g / 1½ cups black pitted
  olives

6 sprigs of fresh oregano,
  leaves removed

olive oil

Add the flour, salt, yeast and sugar to stand mixer and combine with a K beater or dough hook. Add the melted, but slightly cooled, butter, then add the milk and beaten eggs. Add the vinegar, olives and oregano and beat until the dough has a smooth consistency.

Roll out the dough into a long baguette shape and slice it into three strips lengthways, leaving around 2cm / ¾in at the top of the dough so that the three strips are still connected. Plait the dough then connect the ends so you have a plaited circle.

Transfer to either an oiled baking tray (pan) or an oiled casserole dish and allow to prove for around 45 minutes. Preheat the oven to 220°C / 425°F / gas mark 7.

Brush a little milk or water over the top of the loaf and bake for 15 minutes before reducing the temperature to 200°C / 400°F / gas mark 6, and cooking for a further 15–20 minutes or until golden.

The loaf is done once it is golden and hollow sounding when tapped. Cool on a wire rack.

Walnut & Raisin Loaf

SERVES 4–6

5 eggs

3 tbsp coconut oil, melted

2 tbsp honey

260g / 2½ cups ground almonds

1 tsp GF baking powder

½ tsp ground cinnamon

sprinkle of sea salt flakes

130g / 1 cup walnut halves, toasted

70g / ½ cup raisins

butter, to serve

Preheat the oven to 180°C / 360°F / gas mark 4. Line a 25cm (10in) loaf tin (pan) with parchment paper.

Break the eggs into a large bowl. Add the melted coconut oil and honey, whisking to ensure everything is thoroughly mixed.

Add the ground almonds, baking powder, cinnamon and salt, then add the toasted walnuts and raisins. Mix together well.

Pour the mixture into the lined loaf tin (pan). Bake for around 30–35 minutes or until golden.

Remove from the oven and allow to cool slightly before turning out of the tin. Serve warm, sliced, with butter.

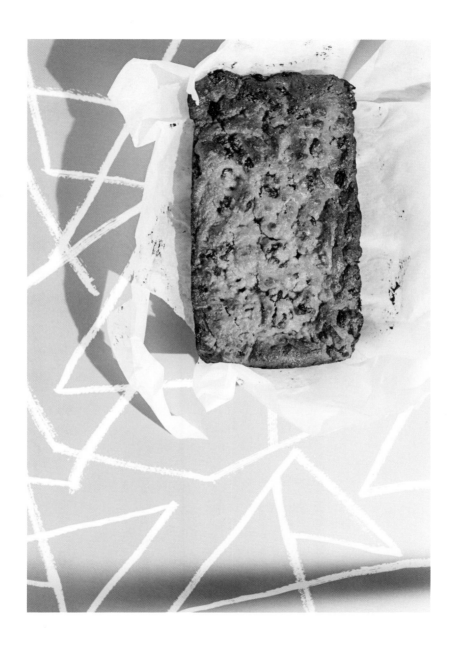

Make friends with gluten-free flour

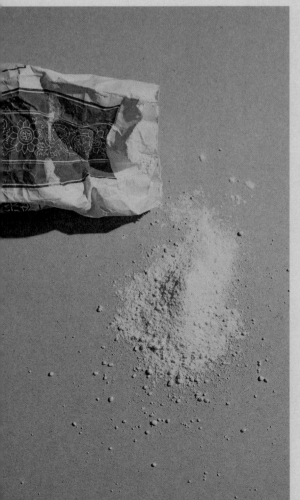

Rice Flour

Great for making pasta, noodles and pancakes. White rice flour is widely available – you have to work a bit harder to find brown rice flour (try health food shops), but it's far healthier.

Chickpea / Gram Flour

High in fibre and a go-to in Indian cooking as it's perfect for rustling up flatbreads. Also use in batters to coat ingredients before frying – it's gives a lovely crispy finish.

Ground Almond / Almond Flour

You can find very finely ground almond packaged as flour, though anything labelled 'ground almonds' works just as well. It's ideal for baking cakes, muffins, macarons, tart cases and biscuits (cookies) and has a mild, nutty flavour.

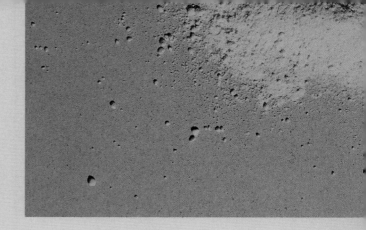

Oat Flour

When made with uncontaminated oats, oat flour is gluten free – which is lucky, as it gives a lovely rich, nutty flavour to bakes, breads, muffins and loaf cakes. It holds moisture well, which is vital in baking, and also gives cookies extra chewiness. Always check the label.

Coconut Flour

This is dried and ground coconut meat. It's a saviour in bread and cake baking, however it doesn't hold moisture very well and can result in a dry bake, so counteract this with lots of wet ingredients.

Quinoa Flour

A great option for bread making, brownies and pancakes. It also has a high protein content.

Buckwheat Flour

Don't be put off by the 'wheat' part of buckwheat. This is actually an easy, go-to, gluten-free substitute for plain (all-purpose) white flour. It's also high in antioxidants: bonus.

Tapioca Flour

Tapioca comes in the form of pearls, flakes, starch and flour, which means there are a variety of ways to use it and it's another great alternative to plain (all-purpose) white flour. It works as a thickening agent in sauces and soups, and for making pudding-like desserts.

Teff Flour

Gently nutty and very good for you compared to plain (all-purpose) flour (it is high in iron and protein), teff works well in baking. It's an ancient grain and best known as the key ingredient in Ethiopian flatbreads.

Banished bread, but still suffering? The culprit might be the toaster. This humble, communal device is the ultimate gluten collector. Go old school and pop your GF bread under the grill — just don't forget to set a timer!

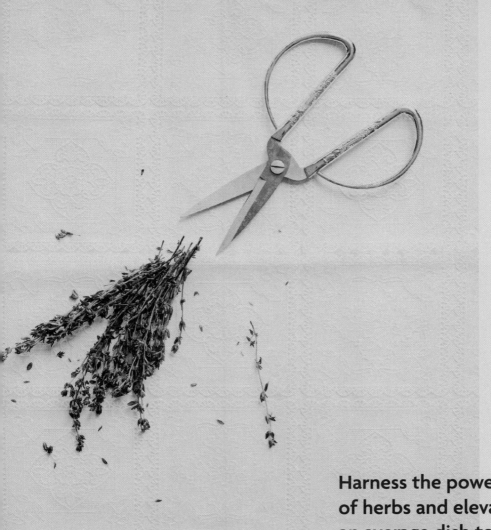

Harness the power of herbs and elevate an average dish to higher heights. You can infuse oils (pages 81–83), make nifty, tasty butters (page 84) or use as a fresh topping.

Confit Cherry Tomatoes, Garlic or Shallots

MAKES 1 LARGE JAR

BASE MIXTURE

550ml / 2½ cups olive oil

1 bulb garlic, cloves peeled

5 sprigs of fresh rosemary
  or thyme

2 fresh bay leaves

generous sprinkle of sea salt
  flakes

1 tbsp black peppercorns,
  roughly ground

rind of ½ lemon, pared

CONFIT CHERRY TOMATOES

5–6 large vines of good
  quality cherry tomatoes

CONFIT GARLIC

5 bulbs garlic, peeled

CONFIT SHALLOTS

400–500g / 14–17½oz baby
  (round) shallots, peeled

First, make the base mixture – this allows you to confit either the tomatoes, garlic or shallots, or you can scale up the base mixture ingredients and make enough for a jar of each.

Begin by pouring the oil into a medium heavy-based saucepan or casserole dish. Place over a low heat. Next place your garlic, herbs, seasoning and lemon into the oil.

Once the oil is hot, but not boiling, add the cherry tomato vines or garlic or shallots, reduce the heat and allow to simmer for 20–25 minutes, either until the tomato skins are wrinkled and soft, or the garlic or shallots are softened.

Remove from the heat, allow to cool, then transfer the contents of the pan to a sterilized jar.

These will keep for around a month – store in a cool place or keep in the fridge.

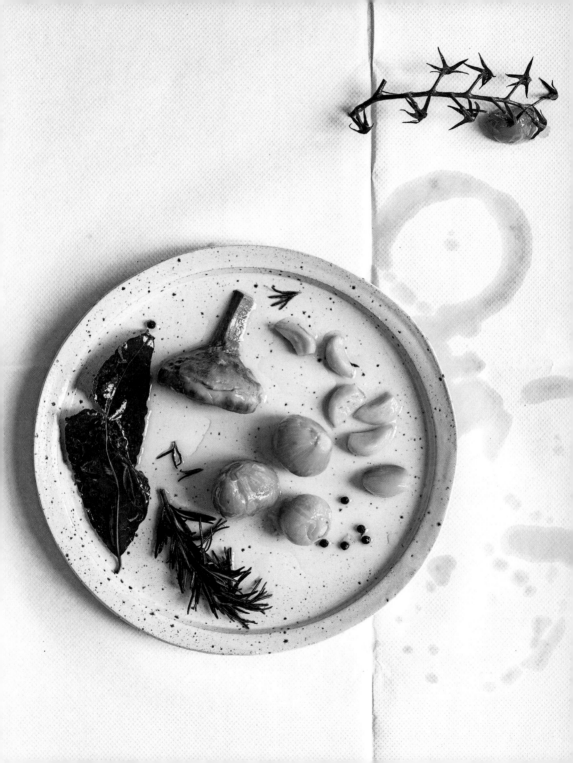

Confit Artichokes

MAKES 1 LARGE JAR
550ml / 2½ cups olive oil
1 bulb garlic, cloves peeled
5 sprigs of fresh thyme
2 fresh bay leaves
generous sprinkle of sea salt
  flakes
1 tbsp black peppercorns,
  roughly ground
1 whole lemon, plus the rind
  of ½ lemon
10 large globe artichokes

Begin by pouring the oil into a medium heavy-based saucepan or casserole dish. Place over a low heat. Next place your garlic, herbs, seasoning and lemon rind into the oil so they can begin to confit while you prepare the artichokes.

Fill a large bowl with cold water. Cut the lemon in half, squeeze the juice into the water, then add the shells to the water too.

Peel off the outer leaves of an artichoke until you reach the lighter, paler leaves. Now trim across the top of the artichoke, leaving around 2.5–4cm / 1in –1½in of artichoke. Take a vegetable peeler and trim around the base and stem, removing any fibrous pieces and neatening it up.

Now cut the artichoke in half down the stem, and cut out and discard the 'choke' – any of the fluffy, fibrous pieces that remain in the centre.

Transfer the prepared artichoke immediately to the bowl of lemon water. This will prevent it from oxidizing and the flesh from darkening. Prepare all the artichokes in the same way.

Add the artichoke halves to the oil, increase the temperature and when small bubbles begin to form around the artichokes reduce the heat again. Allow to confit over a low heat for around 15–20 minutes or until soft but not mushy. Cover with parchment paper to avoid any bits sticking out of the oil.

Once cooked allow to cool, then transfer the artichokes and their oil to a sterilized jar. They will keep for a month.

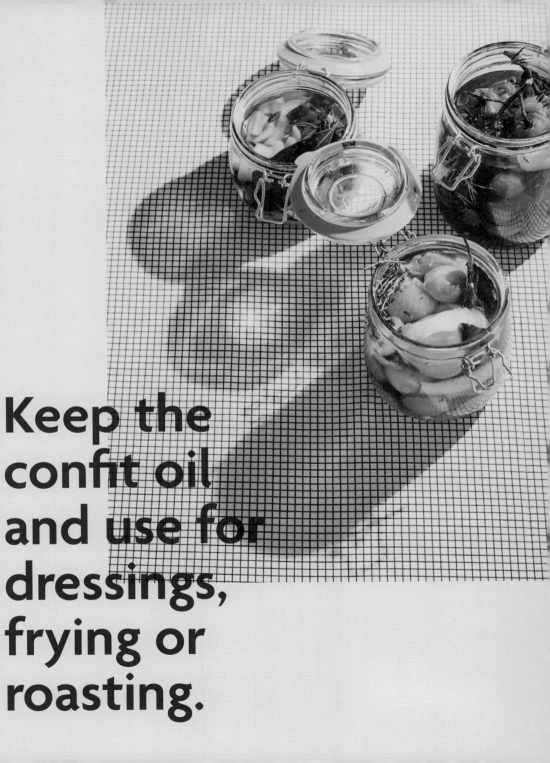

Keep the confit oil and use for dressings, frying or roasting.

Piccalilli

1 large head of cauliflower, cut into small florets (use the stem, too, cubed)

300g / 10½oz green beans, roughly chopped

2 green chillies, finely sliced

15 baby shallots, peeled and quartered

2 small cucumbers, cut in half lengthways, halved again and cut into chunks

200g / 1½ cups sea salt flakes

2 heaped tbsp ground cumin

2 tbsp mustard seeds

2 tbsp ground turmeric

1 tbsp ground black pepper

2 tbsp English mustard powder

3 tbsp GF plain (all-purpose) flour

300ml / 1¼ cups white wine vinegar

3 tbsp caster (superfine) sugar

2 cloves garlic, peeled and finely sliced

3 bay leaves

Begin by preparing all the vegetables: cauliflower, beans, chillies, shallots and cucumbers. Place them in a large bowl, sprinkle over the salt, then pour in enough water to cover everything. Allow to soak for at least 1–2 hours then drain.

For the sauce, combine the cumin, mustard seeds, turmeric, black pepper, mustard powder and flour in a large saucepan, then add the vinegar and sugar and stir into a paste, heating over a medium–low heat. Add several generous splashes of water if it's a little thick. Allow to cook for 2–3 minutes or until the sugar dissolves.

Add the garlic and bay leaves, then add all the salted (and drained) vegetables. Stir to evenly cover with the sauce and cook over a medium heat for around 10–12 minutes.

Divide into sterilized jars, then put the lids on and leave for 4–5 weeks before eating. Store somewhere dry and cool. It will keep for 1–2 months. Once opened, keep refrigerated.

Pickled Onions

MAKES 1 LARGE JAR
or two medium jars
25–30 baby shallots,
  peeled (see Tip)
40g / 3 tbsp salt
1l / 4¼ cups white wine
  vinegar
150g / ¾ cup granulated
  sugar
1 tbsp black peppercorns
  (left whole)
2 tsp coriander seeds
1 bay leaf
½ red chilli, finely sliced

**/ To easily remove the
shallot skins, cover with
boiling water, leave for
10 minutes and then rub
the skins off.**

Place the shallots in a bowl, cover with the salt and leave overnight.

Rinse the shallots, then pat dry with kitchen paper.

Heat the vinegar, sugar, spices, bay leaf and chilli with 800ml / 3½ cups water over a medium heat until the sugar dissolves. Avoid bringing the liquid to the boil.

Place the shallots into sterilized jars and pour the warm vinegar over until they're completely covered, adding in the peppercorns and spices too. Seal and allow to pickle for around 3–4 weeks before eating. Store in a dry and cool place while pickling.

Refrigerate after pickling and opening. The onions will keep for 1–2 months.

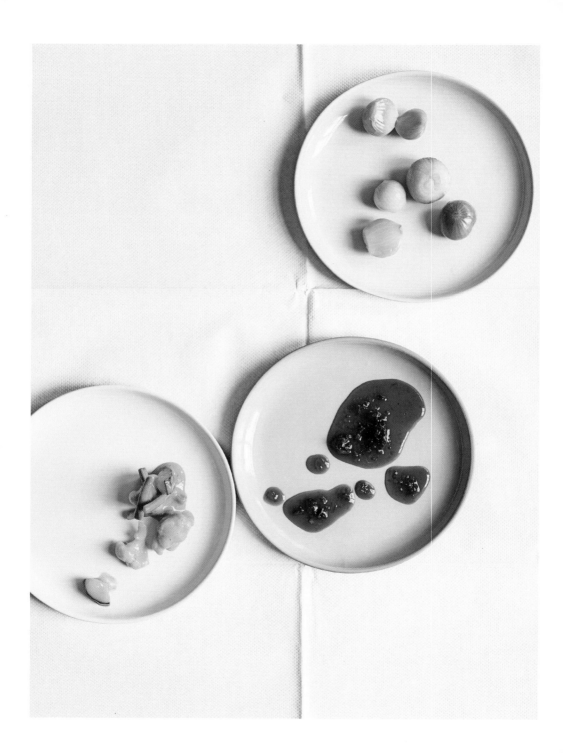

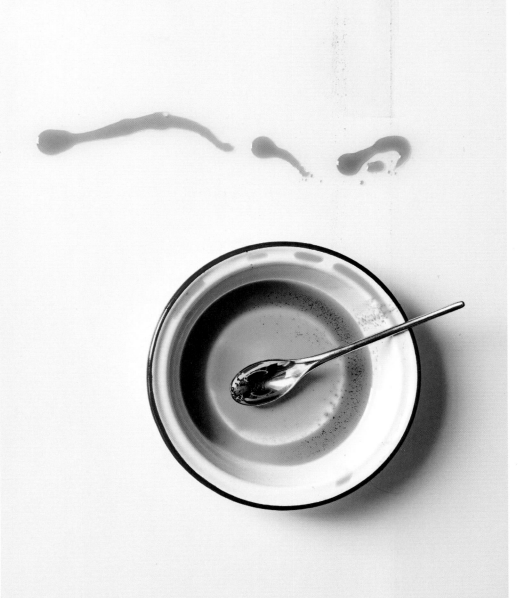

Sticky Chilli Jam

MAKES 2–3 SMALL JARS

5 red chillies, deseeded and
  roughly chopped

2.5cm / 1in piece of fresh root
  ginger, peeled and roughly
  chopped

1 onion, diced

3 cloves garlic, peeled

450g / 2¼ cups golden caster
  (superfine) sugar

100ml / generous ⅓ cup
  apple cider vinegar

Blitz together the chillies, ginger, onion and garlic along with 100ml / ⅓ cup water in a food processor until the ingredients are finely chopped.

Next, put the chilli mixture in a pan along with the sugar and vinegar and cook over a medium heat for 3–4 minutes, until the sugar dissolves.

Increase the heat and bring the mixture to a boil. Once boiling, reduce the heat again and allow to simmer for around 20–25 minutes or until sticky and jam-like.

Carefully spoon the hot jam into hot sterilized jars, seal and set aside to cool. Once opened, keep in the refrigerator and use within 1 month.

Herb Oils

PARSLEY, LEMON
& BLACK PEPPER OIL

large bunch of fresh flatleaf
    parsley, leaves picked from
    stems
generous pinch of sea salt
    flakes
1 tsp freshly ground black
    pepper
zest and juice of ½ lemon
250ml / 8½fl oz rapeseed
    (canola) oill

60–100cm / 24–40in piece
    of thin-weave muslin
    (cheesecloth)

CORIANDER & JALAPEÑO OIL

large bunch of fresh
    coriander (cilantro), leaves
    picked from stems
generous pinch of sea salt
    flakes
zest and juice of 1 lime
1 jalapeño pepper, end
    removed and quartered
250ml / 8½fl oz rapeseed
    (canola) oil

60–100cm / 24–40in piece
    of thin-weave muslin
    (cheesecloth)

Decide which herb oil you're making. Blitz all the ingredients for that oil in a food processor until you have a smooth consistency. Taste and adjust the seasoning to your preference.

Transfer to a saucepan and bring to the boil over a high heat, whisking the entire time. Allow to boil for 2 minutes – it should be a vibrant green colour.

Fill a shallow dish with iced water and sit a metal bowl in the water. Pass the oil through a sieve (strainer) lined with the muslin (cheesecloth), into the metal bowl. This will ensure that it cools down quickly.

Transfer the oil to a sterilized airtight glass bottle. It will keep for 2–3 months.

Mint Oil

MAKES 250ML
generous 1 cup

large bunch of fresh mint,
  leaves picked from stems
zest and juice of 1 lime
250ml / 8½fl oz rapeseed
  (canola) oil
salt and freshly ground
  black pepper

60–100cm / 24–40in piece
  of thin-weave muslin
  (cheesecloth)

Blitz all the ingredients in a food processor until you have a smooth consistency. Taste and adjust the seasoning to your preference.

Transfer to a saucepan and bring to the boil over a high heat, whisking the entire time. Allow to boil for 2 minutes – it should be a vibrant green colour.

Fill a shallow dish with iced water and sit a metal bowl in the water. Pass the oil through a sieve (strainer) lined with the muslin (cheesecloth), into the metal bowl. This will ensure that it cools down quickly.

Transfer the oil to a sterilized airtight glass bottle. It will keep for 2–3 months.

Even the plainest dish can become a culinary marvel with a drizzle of punchy oil.

MAKES 1 LARGE BOTTLE

around 1 litre / 4¼ cups

ROSEMARY & THYME OIL

6–8 sprigs of fresh rosemary
and thyme

1l / 4¼ cups olive oil

CHILLI OIL

6 birds' eye chillies (for extra
heat prick the chillies but
leave whole)

3–4 tsp dried chilli flakes,
to taste

1l / 4¼ cups olive oil

SMOKED GARLIC OIL

1 bulb smoked garlic, cloves
peeled but left whole

1 tbsp black peppercorns

1 bay leaf

1l / 4¼ cups olive oil

Infused Oils

Decide which flavoured oil you're making and place the flavouring ingredients in a sterilized glass bottle.

Gently heat the olive oil to around 75°C / 165°F, so it's hot but not boiling, then pour it over the flavourings in the bottle.

Seal the bottle and leave to infuse for around a month in a cool, dark place.

The oil should be used within around 3 months.

Herb Butters

MAKES 200G / 7OZ

BASIL BUTTER

30g / 1oz fresh basil

sprinkle of sea salt flakes or
  smoked sea salt flakes

zest of ½ lemon (optional)

200g / ¾ cup plus 2 tbsp
  good-quality butter, at room
  temperature

SMOKED SALT
& THYME BUTTER

30g / 1oz or thyme leaves

sprinkle of sea salt flakes or
  smoked sea salt flakes

zest of ½ lemon (optional)

200g / ¾ cup plus 2 tbsp
  good-quality butter, at room
  temperature

WILD GARLIC BUTTER

30g / 1oz wild garlic

sprinkle of sea salt flakes or
  smoked sea salt flakes

zest of ½ lemon (optional)

200g / ¾ cup plus 2 tbsp
  good-quality butter, at room
  temperature

Decide which flavoured butter you're going to make. If you're making the basil or thyme butters, remove the leaves from the stalks. Muddle the herbs of your choice or garlic with a pestle and mortar with the sea salt flakes and lemon zest, if using.

Thoroughly combine the muddled herbs or garlic with the soft butter, then place on a large rectangle of cling film (plastic wrap).

Wrap, then roll the butter into a long even tube, before chilling or freezing. It will keep for a couple of weeks in the fridge or around 6 months if frozen. Defrost in the fridge before use.

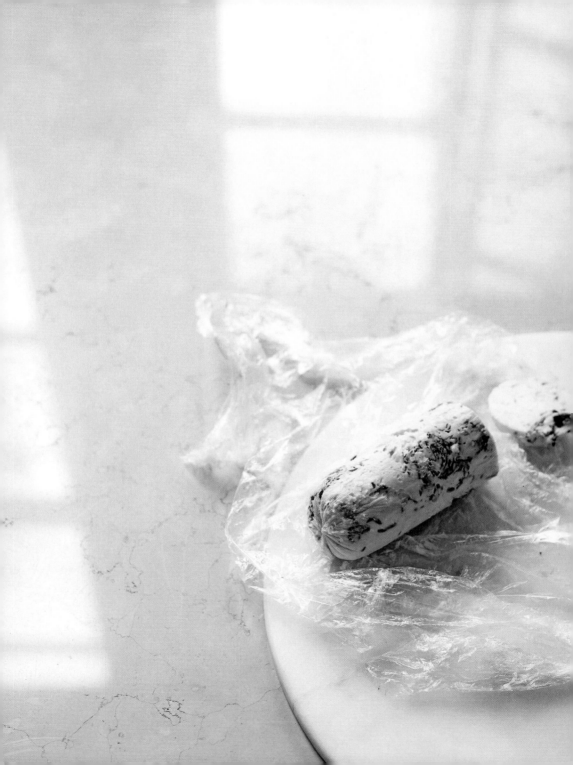

Calamari Rings / Crispy Sage Leaves with Truffle Honey

SERVES 4–6

BATTER

150g / 1 cup plus 2 tbsp self raising (self-rising) flour
225ml / scant 1 cup chilled sparkling water
sprinkle of sea salt flakes
zest of ½ lemon

CALAMARI RINGS

1l / 4¼ cups vegetable oil
3 medium-sized squid, around 120g / 4¼oz each, cut into rings around 5mm / ¼in thick
2 kaffir lime leaves, very finely sliced
1 green chilli, finely sliced
2 spring onions (scallions), finely sliced
sprinkle of sea salt flakes

CRISPY SAGE LEAVES

3 bunches of fresh sage, left as stalks
enough vegetable oil to fully cover the sage leaves
sprinkle of sea salt flakes
truffle honey (optional)

Whisk together the batter ingredients in a bowl until you have a smooth consistency. Place in the fridge.

Heat the oil in a large saucepan to around 180°C / 360°F. Check the temperature by placing a small chunk of bread in the oil – it should fizz immediately and float to the top when the oil is hot enough.

Remove the batter from the fridge. Dip the calamari rings in the batter then transfer to the hot oil. Don't overload the pan, fry just 5–6 rings at a time. Allow the oil to come back up to temperature before doing the next batch.

Once crisp and almost golden, after around a minute or so, remove the calamari from the oil with a slotted spoon and drain on kitchen paper. Transfer to a serving dish, and sprinkle with the lime leaves, chilli, spring onions (scallions) and sea salt. Best served while hot.

For the sage leaves, gently dip the sage leaves in the batter before transferring to the hot oil. For a more delicately battered leaf, give each stalk a gentle shake before transferring to the oil.

Fry 4–5 stalks at a time using the method above. Once crisp and almost golden, after around a minute, remove from the oil with a slotted spoon and drain on kitchen paper. Sprinkle with salt and serve with a drizzle of truffle honey.

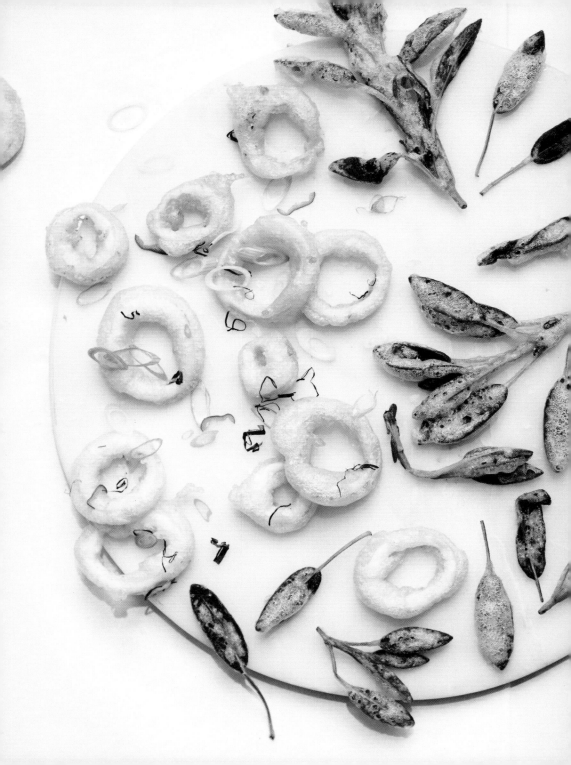

Corn Chips
/ Thyme Salt

SERVES 4–6

4 corn tortillas, cut into
  bite-sized triangles

drizzle of oil

THYME SALT

1 tbsp sea salt flakes

6 sprigs of fresh thyme,
  leaves removed

Preheat the oven to 190°C / 375°F / gas mark 5.

Place the tortilla triangles on a non-stick baking tray (pan)
or line the tray with parchment paper first.

Drizzle with a little oil, then roast until golden – around
10–12 minutes.

For the salt, simply muddle together the thyme leaves and
the sea salt flakes. Once combined, sprinkle over the corn
chips while they're still warm.

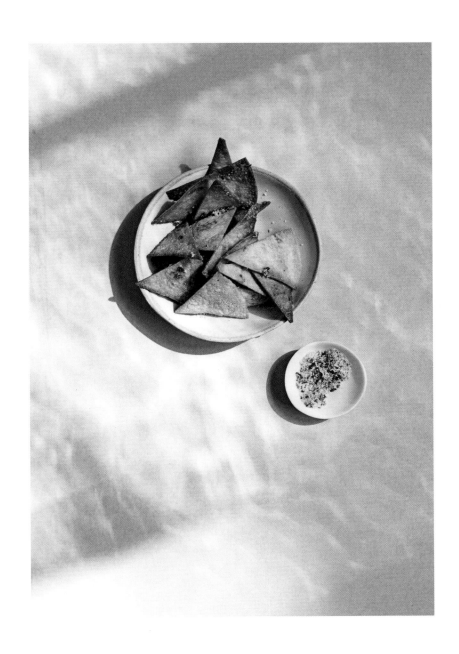

Tapioca & Squid Ink Crackers

SERVES 4–8

150g / 1 cup tapicoa (small
 pearls)
7g / ¼oz sachet of squid ink
1l / 4¼ cups vegetable oil,
 plus extra for brushing
sea salt flakes
Sticky Shallot Hummus and
 Guacamole (see opposite),
 to serve

Preheat the oven to 150°C / 300°F / gas mark 2.

Bring a medium pan of water to the boil and add the
tapioca pearls. Whisk continuously until they begin to float
to the top of the water. Reduce the heat and allow to cook
for around 12 minutes, stirring every now and then to
ensure they don't stick. Remove the pan from the heat but
let the tapioca continue to cook for 5–10 minutes more,
or until the centres become clear and no longer white.

Next, pass the tapioca through a sieve (strainer),
discarding any excess liquid, then rinse the pearls to
remove the starch, and drain. Transfer the drained tapioca
to a bowl and add the squid ink. Mix together.

Line a baking tray (pan) with parchment paper, then
brush on a little extra oil to avoid any possibility of
sticking. Spoon over an even, thin layer of tapioca and
place the tray in the oven.

Allow to dry out completely for around 2–3 hours. Once
cooked, remove from the oven, and roughly break into
chunks around 7.5cm / 3in.

Heat the vegetable oil in a large saucepan and fry the
tapioca pieces in batches until they puff up. Remove from
the oil with a slotted spoon and drain on kitchen paper.
Sprinkle with a little sea salt and allow to cool.

Serve with Sticky Shallot Hummus and Guacamole.

Guacamole

SERVES 4–6

2 cloves garlic, peeled

generous pinch of sea salt
  flakes

½ green chilli, finely diced

2 very ripe avocados

juice of 2 limes, plus extra
  if needed

½ small red onion, finely
  diced

several sprigs of fresh
  coriander (cilantro),
  roughly chopped

drizzle of rapeseed (canola)
  or olive oil

Muddle the garlic with the sea salt flakes with a pestle
and mortar, then add the chilli and continue to muddle
until you have a smooth paste. You can also blitz all the
ingredients in a food processor, if you prefer.

Next, add your ripe avocados and mush it all together
until you have a rough/semi-smooth consistency. Add the
lime juice and red onion and finish with the coriander
(cilantro) and a drizzle of oil. Mix together.

Serve immediately or add a little extra lime juice to the
top of the guacamole to stop it darkening. Store in the
fridge and serve when ready.

Sticky Shallot Hummus

SERVES 4–6

400g / 14oz can chickpeas
  (garbanzos)

juice of 1 lemon

3 tbsp tahini (sesame paste)

2 cloves of garlic, peeled

generous pinch of sea salt
  flakes

several glugs of olive oil

2 banana shallots, finely
  sliced into rings

2 sprigs of fresh thyme,
  leaves picked

Add the chickpeas (garbanzos) with a splash of their
water, lemon juice and tahini to a food processor first,
then add the garlic and salt. This helps to avoid any
ingredients sticking to the sides. Blitz on the highest
setting until you have a smooth consistency.

Heat the oil in a large frying pan, then add the sliced
shallots and thyme. Allow to cook over a medium heat for
5–6 minutes until the shallots turn translucent, sticky and
a little golden. Add the shallots to the hummus in the food
processor and blitz again until completely smooth.

Serve the hummus topped with a good glug of olive oil
and a sprinkle of sea salt flakes.

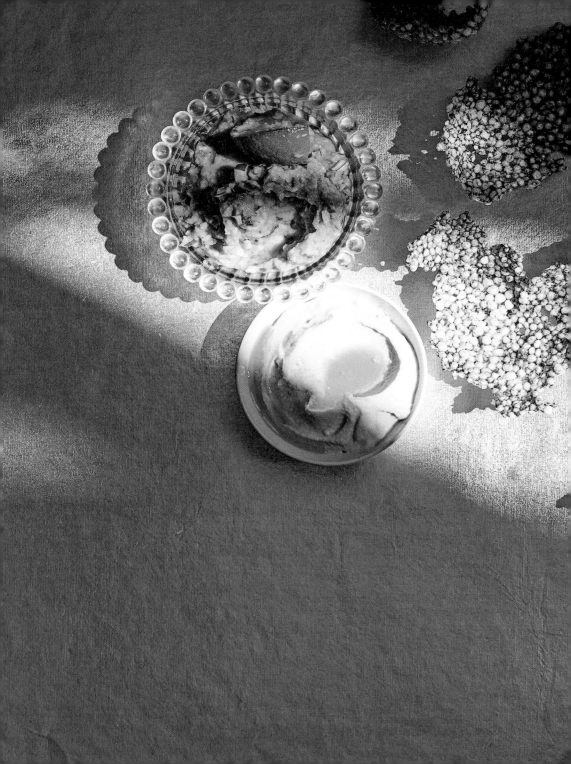

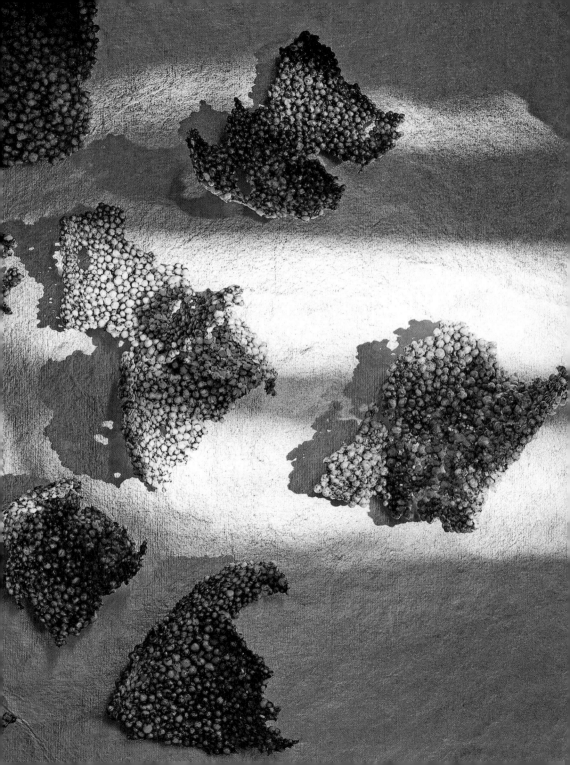

We're living in an age of health-food mania. Interesting grains and unusual snacks (from nut bars to chickpea crisps) are becoming commonplace, and they're often gluten free. Take advantage. Live brave and experiment. Try new things. Say yes!

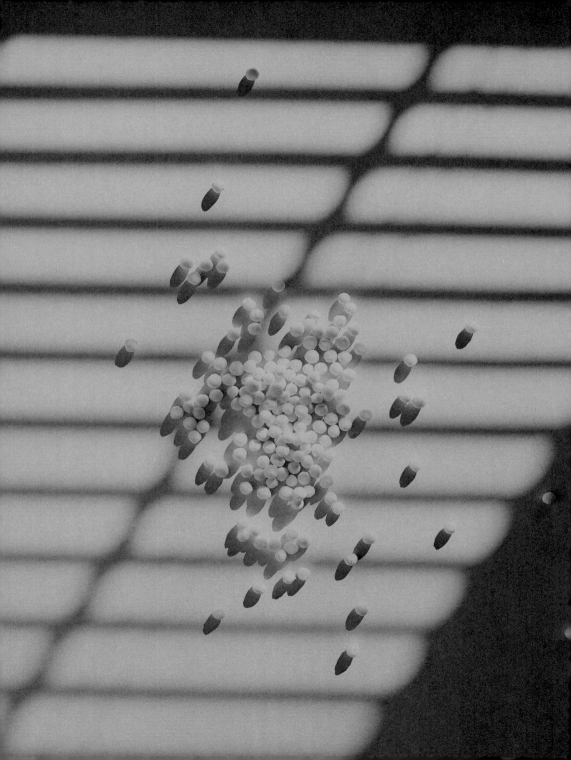

Baba Ganoush / Homemade Flatbreads

SERVES 4–6

4 medium aubergines
  (eggplants)
1 generous tbsp tahini
  (sesame paste)
½ tsp ground cumin
zest of 1 lemon
juice of 2 lemons
several generous glugs of
  good-quality extra virgin
  olive oil
2 tbsp zahter in oil
small bunch of fresh parsley,
  finely chopped
salt and freshly ground
  black pepper

FLATBREADS
380g / 3 cups minus 2 tbsp
  GF self-raising (self-rising)
  flour, plus extra for dusting
sprinkle of sea salt flakes
zest of ½ lemon
270ml / 1¼ cups natural
  yoghurt

Preheat your oven 220°C / 425°F / gas mark 7.

Prick each of the aubergines (eggplants) several times with a fork. If you have a gas hob, then use tongs to carefully sit the aubergines over the flame and allow them to blister. This can also be done under a hot grill (broiler). Char the skins for several minutes before turning until all sides are blistered. Place the charred aubergines on a baking tray (pan) and roast in the oven for 15–20 minutes, or until soft.

Once cooked, allow the aubergines to cool slightly, then peel off the skins and place the flesh in a food processor with the tahini (sesame paste), cumin, lemon zest and juice as well as the oil and seasoning to taste. Blitz until all the ingredients are thoroughly combined and no large lumps of aubergine are left. Taste and adjust seasoning to your preference, then stir in the zahter and parsley.

For the flatbreads, combine the flour, salt and lemon zest, then add the yoghurt and 80ml / ⅓ cup water and bring together into a dough. Divide into six pieces, then roll out into rounds around 5mm / ¼in thick. Sprinkle with a little extra flour to help prevent any sticking.

Heat a griddle until almost smoking, then place the rounds on the griddle for around 30–40 seconds on each side or until they puff up. You can also place under the grill (broiler), cooking for around 2–3 minutes on each side, or until golden.

Serve the flatbreads with the baba ganoush.

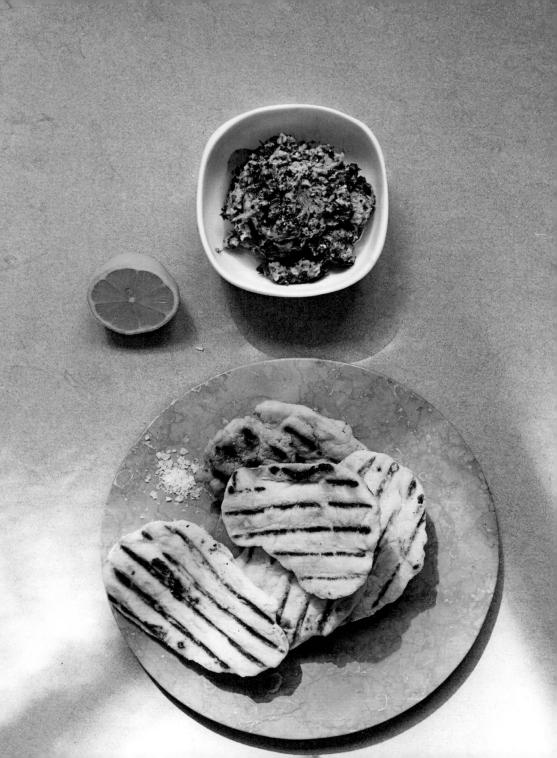

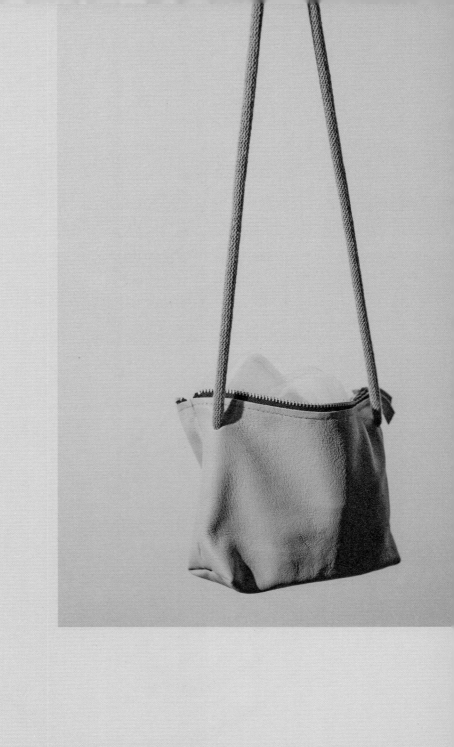

Batch cooking is great, but you might not always want a box of three-bean chilli rattling around in your handbag. Prepare bite-sized, easy-to-carry snacks for emergency hunger pangs and disastrous meals out. Try the balls on page 58, a slice of the nutty loaf on page 62, or even the mini tarts on page 38.

Seabass / Coriander, Lime & Tahini Sauce

SERVES 4

glug of olive or rapeseed
  (canola) oil
around 20 curry leaves
4 fillets of seabass (or any
  sustainable white fish),
  around 200g / 7oz each,
  skin on and pin-boned
several sprigs of fresh
  coriander (cilantro)
zest and juice of ½ lime
salt and freshly ground
  black pepper

CORIANDER, LIME &
TAHINI SAUCE
large bunch of coriander
  (cilantro), leaves picked
  from stems, ends trimmed
2 cloves garlic
½–1 green chilli, to taste
100ml / generous ⅓ cup
  tahini (sesame paste)
80ml / 5½ tbsp freshly
  squeezed lime juice (from
  4–5 limes)

Place the tahini sauce ingredients in a food processor with 150ml / ⅔ cup water and blitz together. Taste and adjust the seasoning to your preference and set to one side.

Add a glug of oil to a large frying pan, heat, then add half the curry leaves, making sure that the oil is hot enough that they fizz immediately. Cook for a minute or so or until they are a vibrant green and crispy. Remove and drain on kitchen paper.

Next, pat the fish fillets dry with kitchen paper and generously season on both sides. Add another good glug of oil to your frying pan (the same one you fried the curry leaves in), place over a medium–high heat and once hot add the fish, skin side down.

Cook for 2–3 minutes or until the skin is golden and crispy. Flip over and cook for another 2–3 minutes on the other side, adding in the remaining curry leaves for flavour. The fish is ready to serve once it's opaque all the way through.

Serve the fish with a generous dollop of the tahini sauce, squeeze over the lime juice and sprinkle over the fried curry leaves, coriander (cilantro) and lime zest.

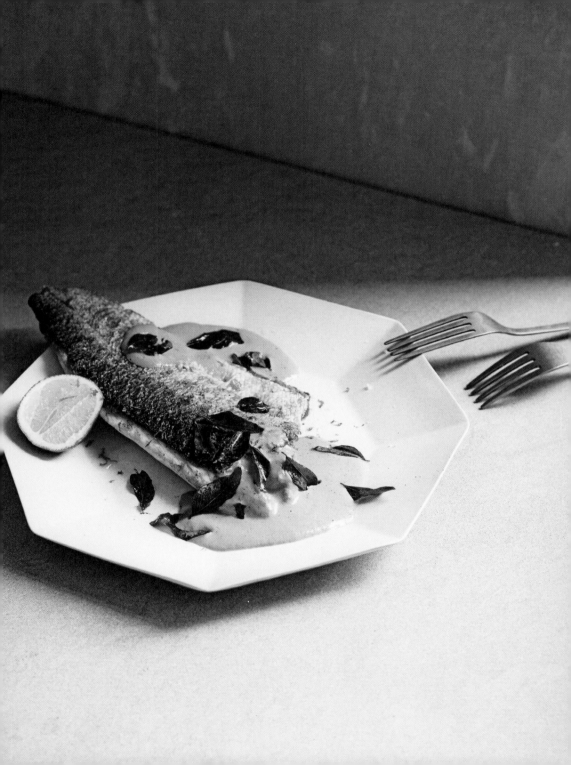

Herbed Ricotta Gnudi / Black Pepper & Parmesan Sauce

GNUDI

50g /1¾oz fresh basil leaves,
  finely chopped
220g / 1 cup ricotta
120g / 3 cups finely grated
  Parmesan
½ fresh nutmeg, finely grated
1 large free-range egg
110g / scant 1 cup
  chickpea (gram) flour, plus
  extra if needed
generous knob of butter
salt and freshly ground
  black pepper

BLACK PEPPER
& PARMESAN SAUCE

200ml / scant 1 cup double
  (heavy) cream
100ml / generous ⅓ cup
  full-fat milk
2 large egg yolks
50g / 1 cup finely grated
  Parmesan, plus extra
  to serve
salt and and freshly ground
  black pepper, to taste

First make the gnudi. Begin by blitzing together the basil leaves and the ricotta in a food processor. Remove from the food processor, transfer to a bowl and add the Parmesan, nutmeg, seasoning and eggs.

Whisk together, adding air to the mixture, before gently folding in the flour. Add a little extra flour if it's still too wet in consistency. It needs to be able to hold its shape and not be too sticky.

Heat the butter in a large frying pan over a medium heat. Use a large tablespoon to spoon generous-sized dumplings into the hot pan. Allow them to cook for 1–2 minutes, turning crispy, then turn. Remove from the pan and drain on kitchen paper. Keep warm.

For the sauce, combine all the ingredients except the Parmesan in a small saucepan and whisk together.

Gently heat over a medium–low heat, stirring constantly for around 3–4 minutes, or until it begins to thicken, then add in the Parmesan. Taste and adjust the seasoning to your preference, adding plenty of black pepper.

Divide the gnudi between four serving bowls, pour over the sauce, and finish with a little extra Parmesan grated over the top.

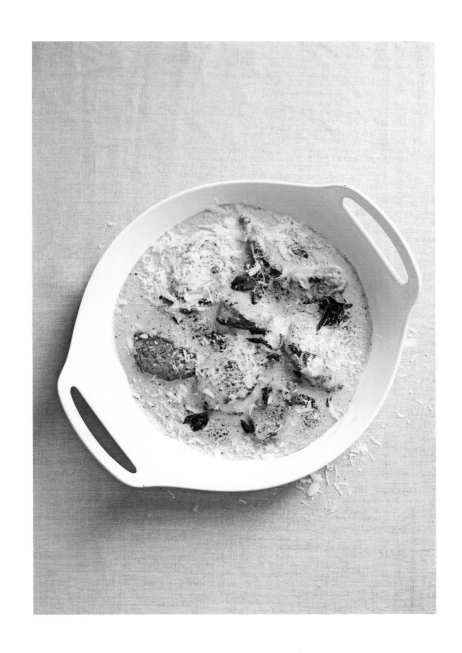

Gochujang BBQ Chicken / Pomelo Spring Green Slaw / Crispy New Potatoes & Fresh Mint

SERVES 4–6

1 free-range corn-fed chicken, around 1.5–1.8kg / 3lb 5oz–4lb
3 tbsp gochujang chilli paste
generous drizzle of sesame oil
2 limes, halved
250ml / 1 cup Korean beer
1.5kg / 3lb 5oz new potatoes
good glug of rapeseed (canola) or olive oil (optional)
generous sprinkle of salt
small bunch of fresh mint, leaves removed from sprigs and roughly chopped

GREEN SLAW

1 head pointed spring greens, finely shredded
small bunch of fresh coriander, ends trimmed
½ pomelo, roughly broken into bite-sized pieces
good dash of white wine vinegar
2–3 tbsp mayonnaise
good sprinkle of sea salt flakes
zest and juice of 1 lime

Preheat oven to 180°C / 360°F / gas mark 4.

Put the chicken in a large roasting tray (pan).

Combine the gochujang paste and sesame oil in a small bowl, then coat the entire chicken with the mixture. Allow the chicken to come to room temperature before cooking. Squeeze the lime halves into the cavity of the chicken, then place the halves inside. >>>

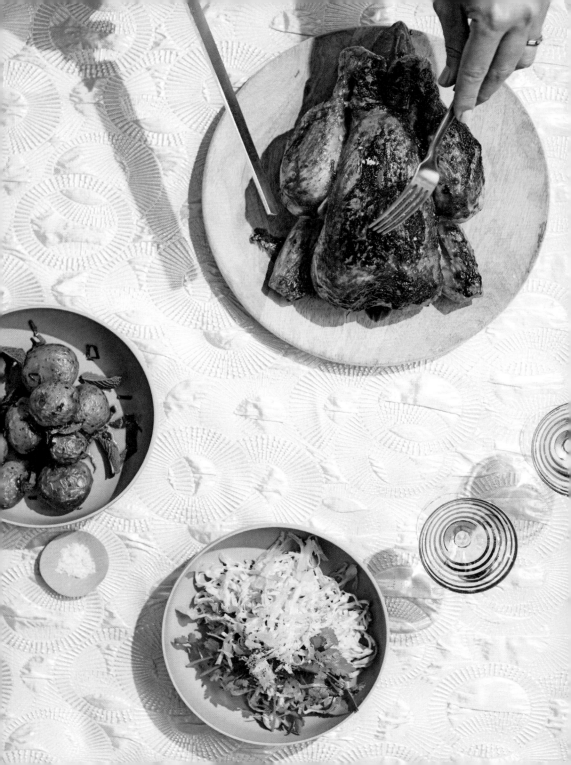

>>> Pour the beer into the tray around the chicken.

Add the new potatoes to the tray, cover with foil and place in the oven and roast for 35 minutes.

Remove the foil and continue roasting for a further 20–45 minutes depending on the size and weight of the chicken. Follow the suggested cooking times but be mindful to not overcook. Sitting the chicken in the beer will help to keep the moisture in and part steam it while in foil.

Once the chicken is cooked, remove from the oven and allow to rest for 15–20 minutes. When the chicken is cooked the skin should be crispy and the meat moist. If you insert a skewer into the thickest part of the thigh, the juices should run clear. Remove the potatoes if they're suitably golden and crisp or, if not, remove the chicken from the tray, crush the potatoes slightly, add a glug of oil, then put them back into the oven to crisp up while the chicken rests.

For the slaw, place the greens, coriander (cilantro) and pomelo in a large bowl. Mix together the vinegar, mayonnaise, salt and lime zest and juice, then pour over the slaw and mix it through so everything is coated. Taste and adjust the seasoning to your preference.

Serve the chicken with the slaw and crispy new potatoes adding a generous scattering of salt and fresh mint over the potatoes.

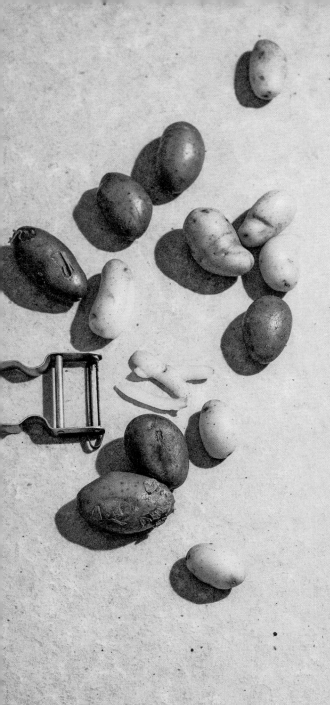

Potatoes come in many, many, shapes and sizes, so don't be fooled by the meagre selection in your supermarket. Go rogue, go local, go to an allotment, plant your own: basically, turf up as many potato varieties as you can, and then fry, roast, boil, steam, mash and more – this is your carb, this is your stodge, and it's delicious.

Roasted Garlic & Taleggio Risotto

SERVES 4

2 small (or 1 large) bulbs
  garlic
good glug of olive oil
large knob of butter
1 onion, finely diced
270g / 1½ cups Arborio rice
good glug of white wine
700–800ml / 3–3½ cups
  vegetable stock
100g / 3½oz Taleggio,
  roughly chopped
generous sprinkle of sea salt

TO SERVE

4 handfuls rocket (arugula)
40g / 1 cup finely grated
  Parmesan
lemon zest
extra virgin olive oil, to
  drizzle

Preheat the oven to 200°C / 400°F / gas mark 6.

Wrap the garlic bulb(s) in foil and roast for 20–25 minutes or until soft.

Start the risotto by adding the olive oil and butter to a saucepan and place it over a medium heat. Once hot, add the onion and cook for around 10 minutes. Next, add the rice and thoroughly stir for 1–2 minutes – don't allow the rice to stick. Now add in the wine and continue to stir.

Once the wine has been absorbed, begin to add the vegetable stock in ladlefuls, allowing the stock to be absorbed each time before adding more. This will take around 20–25 minutes. Check the rice regularly – it should still have a bit of a bite to it, so make sure that it doesn't overcook.

Once all the stock has been absorbed, squeeze in the flesh from the bulbs of roasted garlic and add the chunks of Taleggio, stirring until the cheese is completely melted. Taste and add salt if necessary.

Once the risotto rice has absorbed all the stock and has a good consistency to it (you're aiming for the rice to be slightly al dente and fairly loose) you're ready to serve.

Allow two generous spoonfuls of risotto per person, adding a handful of rocket, a sprinkle of Parmesan, a little lemon zest and an extra drizzle of extra virgin olive oil to each dish.

Brown Butter / Roasted Squash, Smoked Salt Labneh

SERVES 4

1.2kg / 2lb 10oz squash, such
   as Kabocha, acorn,
   butternut or Hubbard,
   quartered

glug of olive oil

generous sprinkle of sea salt
   flakes

several turns of freshly
   ground black pepper

1 sweet potato (approx. 130g
   / 4½oz), peeled into strips

sprinkle of smoked sea
   salt flakes

zest of 1 orange, to serve

SMOKED SALT LABNEH

1 heaped tsp smoked sea
   salt flakes

a sprinkle of freshly ground
   black pepper

250g / 1¼ cups Greek
   yoghurt

HAZELNUT BUTTER

100g / ¾ cup hazelnuts

150g / ⅔ cup butter

sprinkle of smoked sea
   salt flakes

Begin by making the labneh. Stir the smoked salt and
a little black pepper through the yoghurt, then transfer
the mixture to a muslin (cheesecloth) set over a sieve
(strainer). Tie up the muslin and allow to strain for around
1–2 hours, or overnight. It should be the consistency of
cream cheese, or even a little bit more robust. Stored in the
fridge, the labneh will last for 3–4 days.

Preheat your oven to 190°C / 375°F / gas mark 5. Add the
squash quarters to a roasting pan, drizzle with oil and add
seasoning. Roast the pieces of squash for around 25–30
minutes, until they begin to crisp up.

Line a baking tray (pan) with parchment paper or use
a non-stick baking tray. Place the sweet potato strips in
a bowl with a little olive oil and mix so that the strips are
evenly coated in oil. Spread them out on the baking tray,
so none of the strips are overlapping. Roast for around
7–8 minutes until crisp and dry. Remove from the oven,
sprinkle with the smoked salt and allow to cool.

To make the hazelnut butter, spread the nuts out on
a baking tray and roast them in the oven for 3–4 minutes
or until golden. Transfer the hazelnuts to a container with
a lid and shake to remove the skins. Roughly chop the
nuts, leaving a few whole, then combine all the nuts with
the butter in a pan over a low–medium heat, simmering for
4–5 minutes until the butter darkens a little. Season with
smoked salt and keep warm until ready to serve.

To serve, start with the labneh as the base, then add the
squash, drizzle over the hazelnut butter and finish with the
sweet potato crisps, seasoning and orange zest.

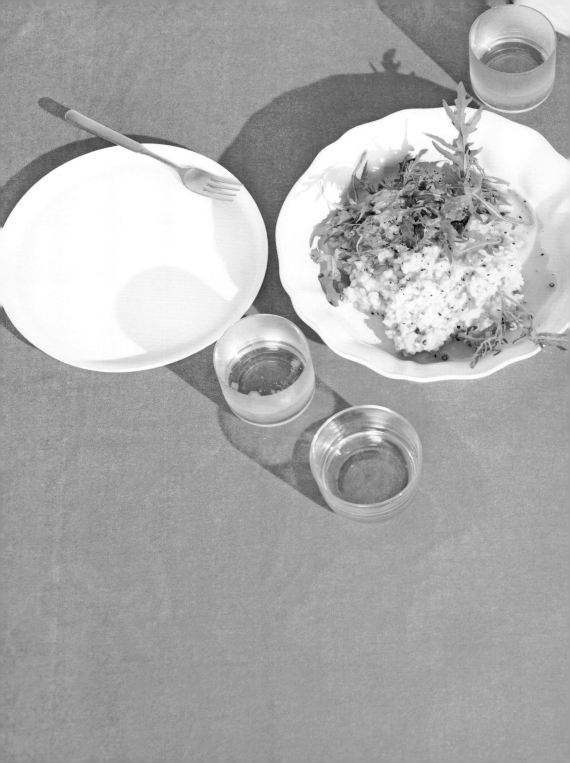

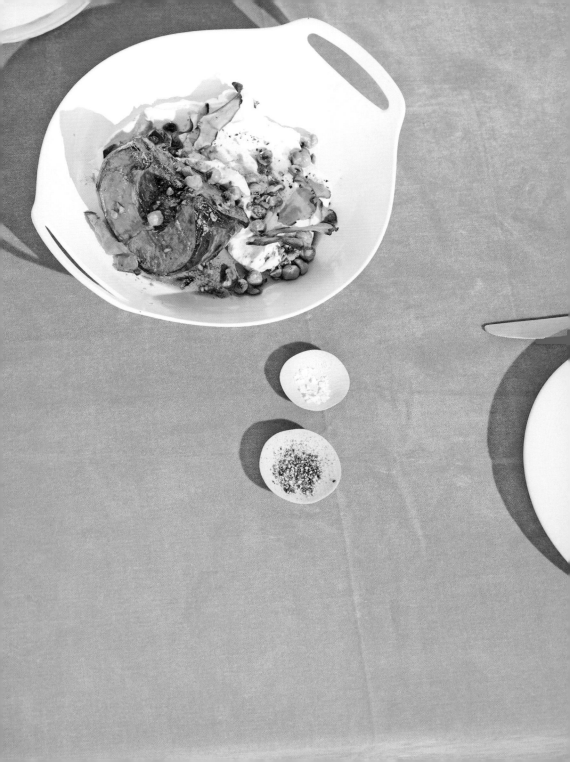

Seafood Stew / Kimchi & Charred Cauliflower Rice

SERVES 4–6

glug of rapeseed (canola) or
   olive oil
1 onion, quartered
2 cloves garlic, crushed and
   roughly chopped
2 stalks lemongrass, ends
   trimmed, bashed and cut
   in half
5cm / 2in piece of fresh root
   ginger, peeled and grated
2 kaffir lime leaves
3 tbsp gochujang chilli paste
250g / 9oz kimchi, plus juice
850ml / 3½ cups seafood
   stock
1 medium head of
   cauliflower, coarsely grated
selection of seafood: 8–12
   king prawns (jumbo
   shrimp), tails left on,
   shell removed; 200g / 7oz
   monkfish, cut into bite-
   sized chunks; 200g / 7oz
   mussels, cleaned
1 lime, quartered

Begin by heating a good glug of oil in a large casserole
dish. Once hot, add in the onion and cook for a couple
of minutes.

Next add in the garlic, lemongrass and ginger, allow to
cook for another couple of minutes before adding in the
lime leaves, Gochujang paste, kimchi (plus juice) and
seafood stock. Allow to cook over a low–medium heat
for 15–20 minutes to allow the flavours to intensify.

Meanwhile, prepare the cauliflower rice. Heat a griddle
pan until almost smoking hot, then add the grated
cauliflower in batches, just briefly charring to add a hint
of smokiness. Set to one side, covering with foil to keep
it warm.

When the cauliflower rice is ready, add the seafood to
the stew, cover and increase the heat. Cook for 2–3
minutes, ensuring that the mussel shells open.

Serve the stew alongside the charred cauliflower rice
with a squeeze of lime over the top.

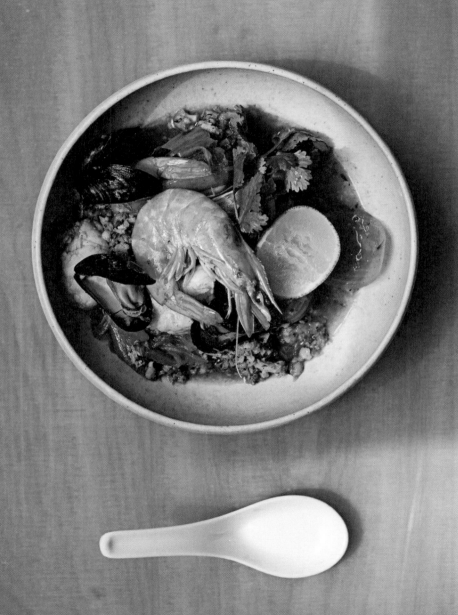

Corn Tacos
/ Fried Fish / Slaw

SERVES 4

4–8 corn tacos

1l / 4¼ cups vegetable oil

500g / 17½oz haddock, cut
  into even bite-size chunks

BATTER

80g / ⅔ cup GF self-raising
  (self-rising) flour

115ml / ½ cup chilled
  sparkling water

sprinkle of sea salt flakes

zest of 1 lime

CORIANDER SLAW

bunch of fresh coriander
  (cilantro)

½ red cabbage, finely sliced

2 tbsp mayonnaise

1 tbsp Sriracha

GARNISH

1 red onion

juice of 1 lime

2 green chillies, finely sliced

2 limes, cut into thirds

Combine all the batter ingredients, whisking until smooth. Store in the fridge until ready to use.

To make the slaw, roughly chop two-thirds of the coriander (cilantro). Place in a bowl with the red cabbage, then refrigerate.

Prepare your garnishes and set to one side. Slice the red onion, squeeze over the lime juice, and store in the fridge until ready to serve.

Warm the tacos, either charring on a hot griddle or heating in a dry non-stick pan for around 30–40 seconds each side. Wrap them in foil and keep warm in an oven preheated to 150°C / 300°F / gas mark 2.

For the fish, heat the vegetable oil to around 180°C / 360°F. Drop a bit of batter in to check the oil is hot enough – it should immediately fizz vibrantly to the top.

Remove the batter from the fridge. Dip the fish pieces in the batter so they are evenly coated. Cook in batches until golden – they will only need 1–2 minutes. Allow the oil to come back up to temperature between batches.

Remove the red cabbage from the fridge, add the mayonnaise and Sriracha and mix well to coat.

Serve everything on a large platter or across a selection of bowls and have everyone make up their own tacos.

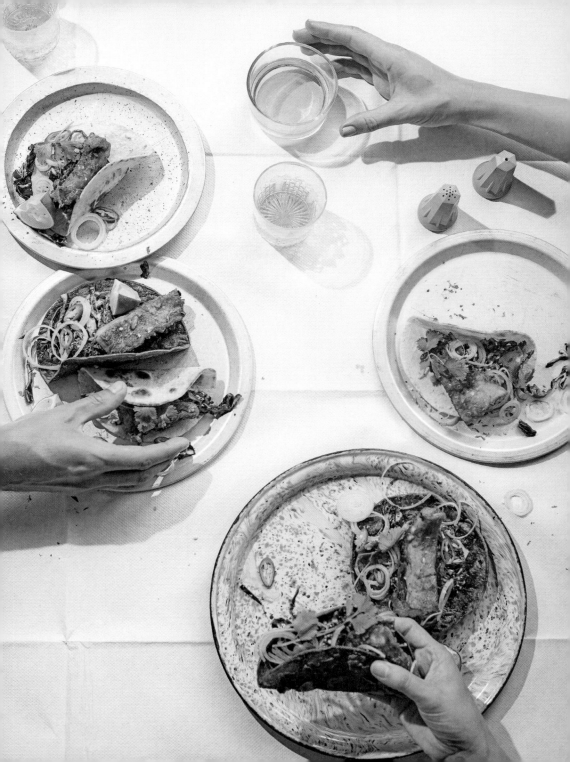

Surf & Turf Paella

SERVES 4–6

1.3l /5½ cups good-quality
    fish stock
generous glug of olive oil
1 onion, finely diced
3 cloves garlic, minced
140g / 5oz spicy chorizo,
    roughly diced
450g / 2¼ cups paella or
    basmati rice
pinch of saffron
1 tsp smoked paprika
100g / ¾ cup frozen peas
8–10 king prawns (jumbo,
    shrimp), shells removed
    (apart from the
    tail) and deveined
200g / 7oz mussels,
    thoroughly cleaned
small bunch of fresh parsley,
    roughly chopped
1 lemon, quartered
salt and freshly ground
    black pepper

Pour the fish stock into a large pan and bring to the boil, before allowing to simmer over a medium heat.

Heat a generous glug of olive oil in a large flat-based dish – ideally a paella dish. Add the diced onion and cook over a medium–low heat for 4–5 minutes or until soft and translucent. Add the garlic and diced chorizo, increase the heat a little, and fry for a few minutes until the chorizo begins to crisp a little.

Add the rice to the pan and evenly coat with all the juices and oil from the chorizo. Sprinkle over the saffron and smoked paprika, then pour in three-quarters of the hot fish stock. Allow to cook over a medium heat for around 15–20 minutes until the majority of the stock has been absorbed. Stir every now and then to stop the rice sticking.

Once the rice is almost done (it should still have a little bite), add the frozen peas, prawns (shrimp) and mussels, plus the remaining stock. Stir and cover with a lid or foil – this will help to cook the mussels – and heat for a further 5–6 minutes or until the mussel shells open (discard any that don't).

Taste for seasoning and adjust to your preference. Serve with a generous sprinkle of chopped parsley, wedges of lemon and a drizzle of oil.

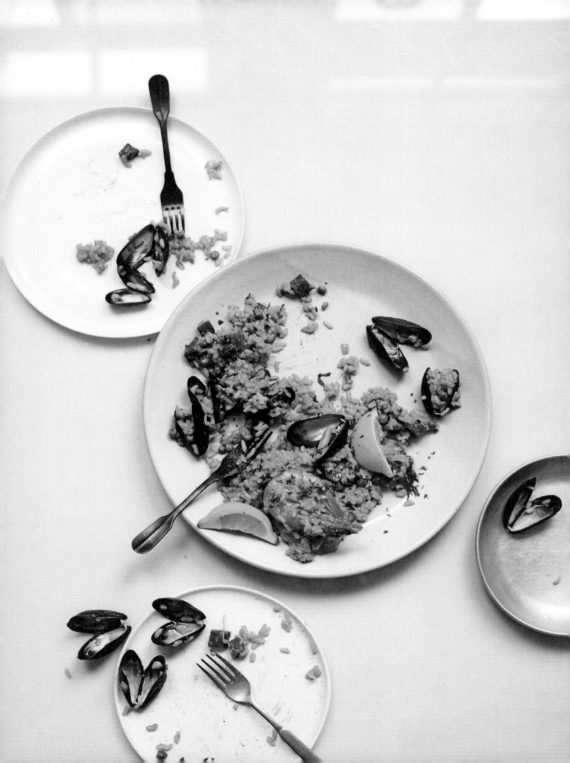

Spiced Pork & Ginger Dumplings / Lemongrass Chicken Broth / Courgetti

SERVES 4

2 green courgettes (zucchini), sprialized

small bunch of fresh coriander (cilantro), ends trimmed

1 green chilli, finely sliced

BROTH

1l / 4¼ cups good-quality chicken stock

2 stalks lemongrass, ends trimmed and bashed

5cm / 2in piece of fresh root ginger, peeled and grated

splash of tamari (optional)

DUMPLINGS

500g / 17½oz good-quality minced (ground) pork

1–2 red chillies, to taste, finely diced

2 cloves garlic, minced

5cm / 2in piece of fresh root ginger, peeled and grated

½ tsp white pepper

generous dash of fish sauce

Begin by combining all the broth ingredients except the tamari in a large saucepan or casserole dish. Bring to the boil, then reduce the heat, cooking for 15–20 minutes while you prepare the dumplings.

Combine all the dumpling ingredients in a bowl, then mush together with your hands and roll the mixture into balls a little smaller than a golf ball. Set to one side until you've rolled all the dumplings, then place them in the broth. Cover with a lid and increase the heat a little, cooking for around 7–8 minutes or until the dumplings are cooked the whole way through.

Taste the broth and adjust the seasoning to your preference, adding a little tamari for extra salt if you need to.

Divide the courgetti up between four serving bowls, then spoon over the broth and divide up the dumplings equally. Serve with a scattering of fresh coriander (cilantro) and sliced chilli.

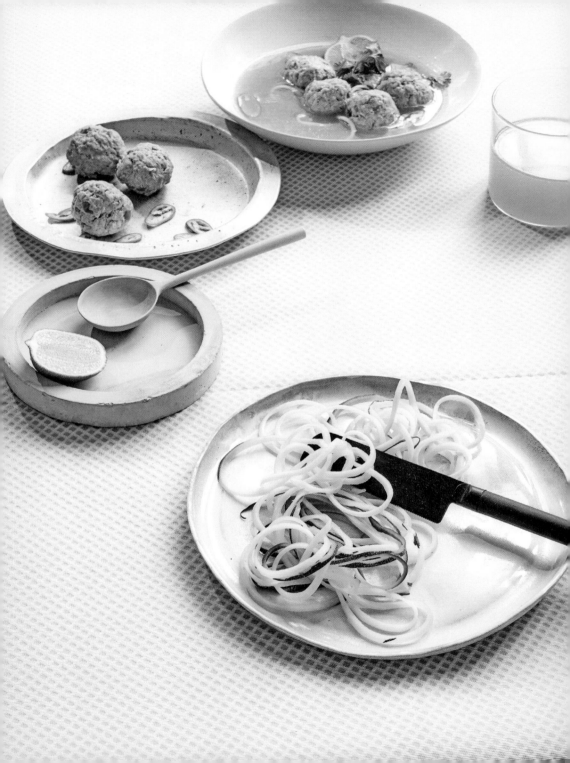

Raid your nearest Asian supermarket and stock your cupboards with delicious gluten-free noodles. They have bite, texture and flavour, and can bulk out a meal in a way that spiralized veg can only dream of.

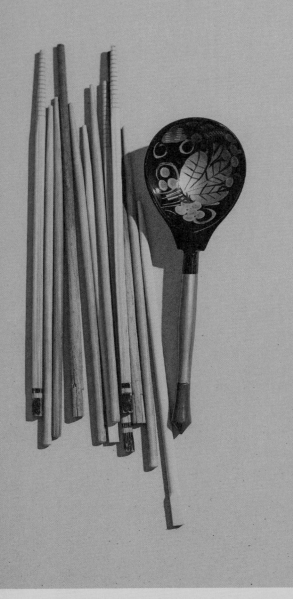

Look out for these (but always check the label):

Soba / made from buckwheat

Shirataki / a plant-based Japanese noodle made from konjac yam

Kelp / these can be vermicelli-like white noodles, or full-on seaweed green

Dang myun / a Korean noodle made from sweet potato

Rice / made from rice and can be vermicelli-like or thin and ribbon-like

Thai Curry / Pork Skewers / Black Rice Noodles

SERVES 4

2 x 400g cans full-fat coconut milk, chilled so that the cream sets at the top of the tin

3 kaffir lime leaves, 1 finely sliced, to garnish

black rice noodles, to serve 4

small bunch of fresh Thai (purple) basil

1 green chilli, finely sliced

2 limes, cut into thirds

PORK SKEWERS

600g / 1lb 5oz pork shoulder, cut into 2cm / ¾in chunks

2 onions, cut into chunks

drizzle of sesame oil

GREEN CURRY PASTE

1 shallot, peeled and roughly chopped

4 large cloves garlic, peeled

5–7.5cm / 2–3in of fresh root ginger or galangal, peeled and roughly chopped

2 stalks lemongrass, ends trimmed, roughly chopped

bunch of fresh coriander (cilantro), stalks plus half of the leaves (the rest can be saved for serving)

3–4 green chillies, to taste

1 tsp ground coriander

½ tsp ground cumin

½ tsp white pepper

3 tbsp fish sauce (optional)

1 tbsp palm sugar or brown sugar

glug of sesame oil

Combine all the green curry paste ingredients in a food processor and blend until you have a smooth paste. This can also be done the traditional way in a large pestle and mortar, starting with the hard ingredients, then adding the softer until you have a smooth paste.

You can make this in advance, cover with more oil and store in the fridge until ready to use. It will keep for between 1–2 weeks. >>>

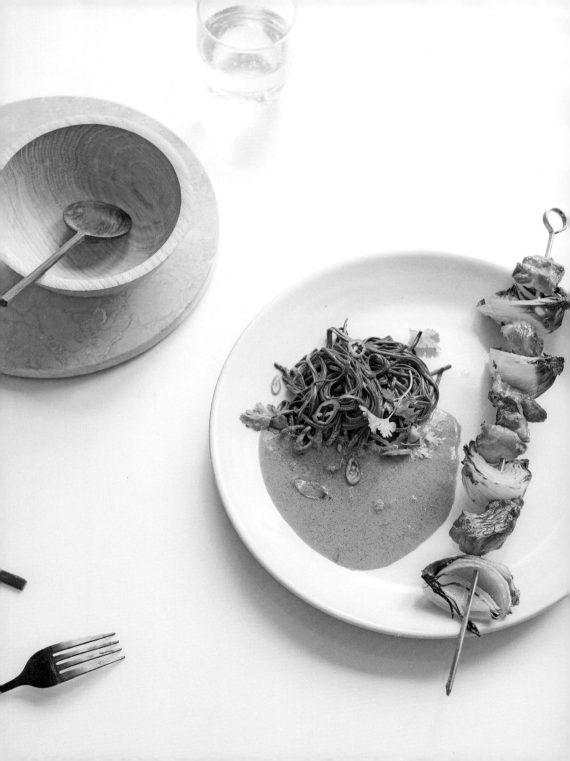

>>> To make the curry, add 4–5 generous dollops of the curry paste to a heavy-based casserole dish or large pan. Allow to cook for 1–2 minutes over a medium–low heat, stirring to prevent any sticking.

Next, scoop out the coconut cream from the top of the chilled cans of coconut milk, add this to the pan, and allow to cook for 2–3 minutes with the curry paste. Now add the remaining coconut milk and whole lime leaves and allow to cook for around 20–25 minutes until the flavour intensifies.

Preheat the grill (broiler) to high.

Thread the pork and onion and pieces alternately onto four skewers, being mindful to not pack the pieces too tight. Drizzle with a little sesame oil and cook them close to the grill (so you get the darker, more charred corners) for around 7–8 minutes. Turn the skewers a few times, so they are evenly cooked.

Prepare the black rice noodles as per the packet instructions, then divide them up across four bowls when ready to serve.

Spoon the Thai green curry sauce over the noodles and divide up the pork skewers.

Scatter over the remaining coriander (cilantro), the sliced lime leaf, Thai basil and sliced green chilli and serve with a good squeeze of lime.

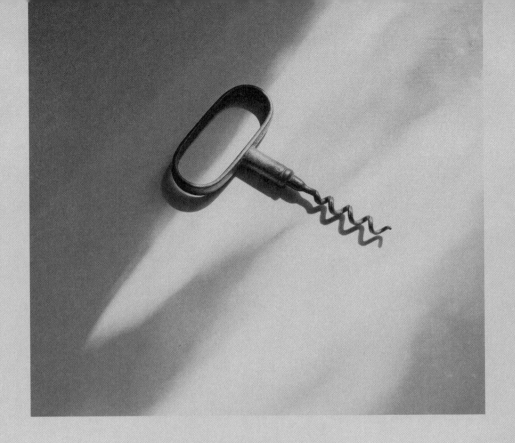

It's a tough break, but beer is pretty much out. You can, however, drown your sorrows in wine, cider and spirits, so that's still most of the bar. If you're heading to a friend's house, take plenty of booze you can drink, and while you're at it, take a bag of corn chips and your own hummus dip (to avoid pitta crumbs in the communal bowl). Yes, it's a faff, but you will be happier drinking your chilled glass of cider and dipping your GF chips, and your friends will be happier knowing they don't have to worry about being the source of your GF-induced pain.

Gluten-free Pasta

SERVES 6
450g (3½ cups) GF white
   bread flour, plus extra
   for dusting
generous pinch of table salt
6 medium eggs (heritage-
   breed free-range eggs give
   a rich yellow yolk)

TO SERVE
your favourite pasta sauce, or
   any of the confit recipes on
   pages 72–74
extra virgin olive oil
finely grated Parmesan
salt and freshly ground
   black pepper

Combine the flour and salt in a large bowl. Whisk the eggs, then combine with the flour until you have a dough. Wrap in clingfilm (plastic wrap) and chill for around 30 minutes in the fridge.

When you remove the dough from the fridge, knead until you have a smooth consistency. It should be a slightly springy ball of dough.

Cut the dough into 6–8 pieces and roll into long, flat strips with a rolling pin before passing through your pasta machine.

Make sure you avoid any sticking by lightly dusting the dough with flour, then pass it through the settings on the pasta machine, starting at the thickest. You will need to pass it through then fold the pasta back over itself and pass it through the same thickness setting several times until the pasta starts to hold together a little better. It may be a little crumbly to begin with, but persevere. I like to only roll down through the first 3–4 settings so that the pasta, when cut into tagliatelle, is a little more robust. It can often help to have an extra pair of hands when passing the pasta through the machine to begin with.

Once prepared, bring a large pan of salted water to the boil and cook the pasta for around 3–6 minutes depending on its thickness.

Serve with your sauce or confit of choice. Finish with a good glug of extra virgin olive oil, seasoning and plenty of grated Parmesan.

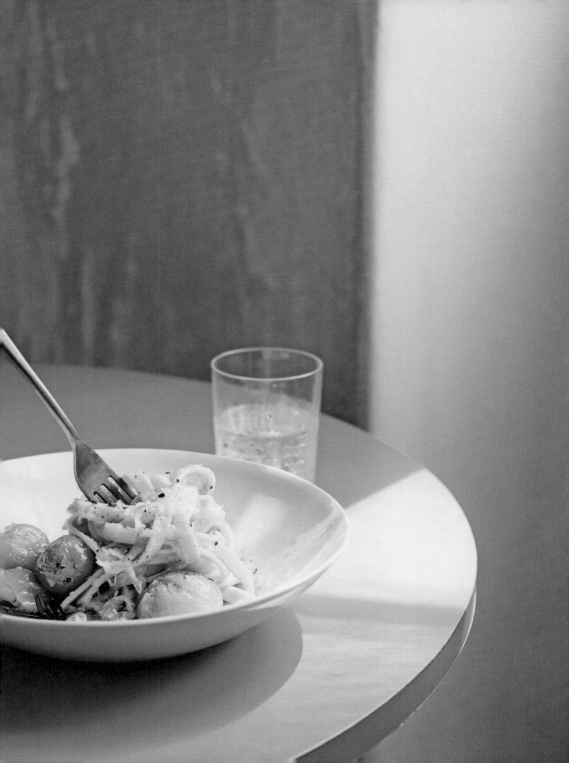

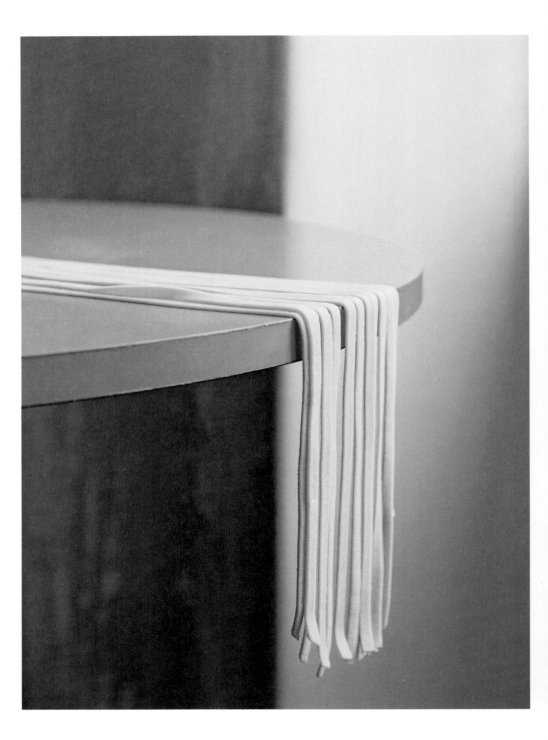

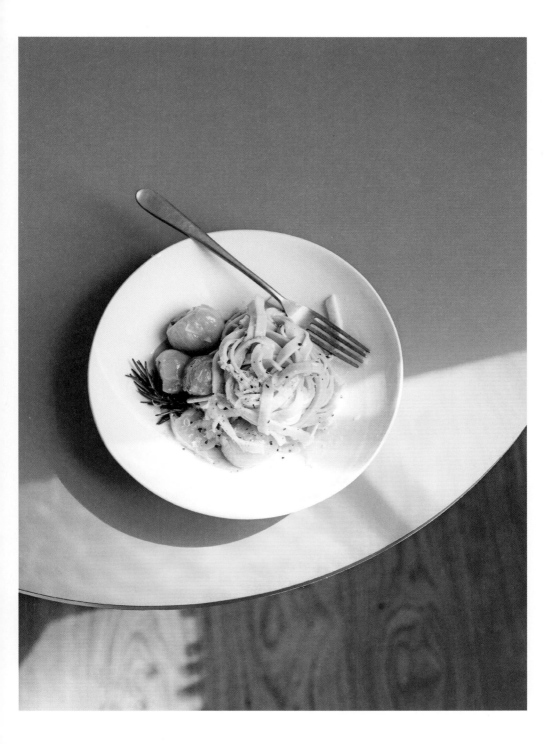

It would be easy to say 'plan ahead, make sure you have plenty of fresh fruit and veg, keep your store cupboard stocked, etc'. But life is good at throwing up trigger situations that an apple simply can't resolve... the drunken night out munchies, the hellish hangover hunger, that intense I'm-crashing-hard-need-cake moment at roughly 4pm each day. The secret to tackling these is having your favourite, delicious snack lined up. For example, have a bag of tortilla chips and a slab of cheese ready at all times – there are few problems that can't be remedied by a plate of nachos. Similarly, a jar of peanut butter, chocolate spread or jam is a handy go-to for a shot of salt, fat and sugar. Ultimately – and this is the tough bit – you need to do your junk-food research: know the snacks you can and can't have, so that when you're in dire need, you can nip to the shop and instantly

triumph.

Ask and you shall (hopefully) get.

Wouldn't it be great if every restaurant was fully prepared for your arrival with a separate kitchen labelled 'gluten free'. Dream, and it will happen! But for now, try a couple of more realistic things. Use social media to follow others in the GF community: make a note of tasty-looking, safe meals they've had out — save yourself the research and follow in their footsteps. If you're stuck, lean on a mainstream chain, which is likely to have at least one GF option on the menu. And if you're visiting an independent, call ahead: explain yourself, ask politely, offer suggestions — a good chef will be happy to experiment. If not, you can vote with your wallet.

Sticky Pineapple Monkfish / Pickled Carrots

\\\\\\\\\\\\\\\\\\\\\\\\\\\\\\\\\\\\\

SERVES 4

300g / 1½ cups sushi rice
2 large carrots, peeled into
   ribbons
glug of white wine vinegar
1 tbsp mirin or honey
2 birds' eye chillies, chopped
2 tbsp gochujang chilli paste
2 cloves garlic, grated
5cm / 2in piece of fresh root
   ginger, finely grated
3 tbsp chopped stem ginger,
   plus 3 tbsp of the syrup
3 glugs of GF tamari
pineapple from half a
   400g/14oz can, cut into
   chunks, juice reserved
1 heaped tsp of Sriracha
good glug of orange juice
small dash of orange food
   colouring (optional)
600g / 1lb 5oz monkfish,
   pinboned and cut into even
   bite-sized chunks

GARNISH

2 tsp sesame seeds
1 red chilli
1 spring onion (scallion)
small bunch of fresh
   coriander (cilantro)
1 lime, sliced into wedges

Begin by cooking the rice as per the pack instructions.

Place the carrot strips in a bowl. Combine a generous glug of vinegar with the mirin or honey and the chillies, then pour over the carrot strips and allow to lightly pickle while you make up the rest of the dish.

Add the gochujang paste, garlic, grated ginger, stem ginger (plus syrup), tamari, pineapple (plus juice), Sriracha and orange juice to a medium-sized frying pan, bring to the boil then reduce the heat and cook over a medium–high heat until you have an almost syrup-like consistency. Add in the orange food colouring, if using.

Prepare the garnishes. Lightly toast the sesame seeds in a dry frying pan over a medium heat until they turn a light golden colour. Slice the chilli and spring onion (scallion) and roughly chop the coriander (cilantro).

Add the monkfish chunks to the sauce in the frying pan and allow to cook over a medium heat. Cook for around 2–3 minutes or until the monkfish is opaque and cooked through.

Serve the rice with a generous portion of the sticky monkfish and pineapple, scatter over the pickled carrot, spring onion, coriander and chilli and serve with lime wedges.

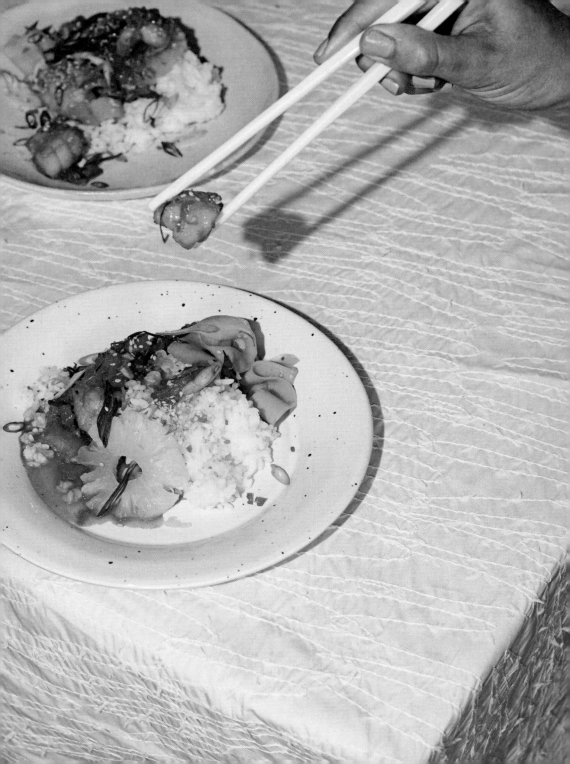

Macaroons
/ Salted Chocolate Dip

//

MAKES 6–10

4 egg whites

135g / 2 cups desiccated
(dried shredded) coconut

145g / 1¾ cups flaked
(slivered) almonds

165g / ¾ cup caster
(superfine) sugar

½ tsp vanilla bean paste

SALTED CHOCOLATE DIP

150g / 5¼oz dark chocolate
(at least 70% cocoa solids),
broken into pieces

½ tsp sea salt flakes, plus
extra for sprinkling

Preheat the oven to 180°C / 360°F / gas mark 4. Line two large baking trays (pans) with parchment paper.

In a heatproof bowl, combine the egg whites, coconut, almond flakes, sugar and vanilla bean paste and set over a pan of boiling water (like a bain-marie). Ensuring the water isn't touching the base of the bowl, stir constantly and cook for around 7–8 minutes or until the egg whites turn opaque.

Next, spoon 6–10 generous dollops of the mixture onto your lined trays, allowing plenty of space between the macaroons.

Bake for 10 minutes at 180°C / 360°F / gas mark 4, then reduce the heat to 170°C / 320°F / gas mark 3 and bake for an additional 10 minutes until golden brown. Once cooked, remove from the oven and allow to cool.

To make the salted chocolate dip, place the chunks of broken chocolate in a bowl over boiling water as before, and allow to melt. Remove from the heat. Add the salt, stir, then dunk the cooled macaroons in the chocolate and place back on the trays to allow the chocolate to set, finishing with a little extra sprinkle of sea salt flakes. Alternatively, simply drizzle the salted chocolate over the macaroons. Serve once the chocolate has set.

/ Store the macaroons in an airtight container and serve the next day with coffee. They will last 2–3 days, stored in the fridge.

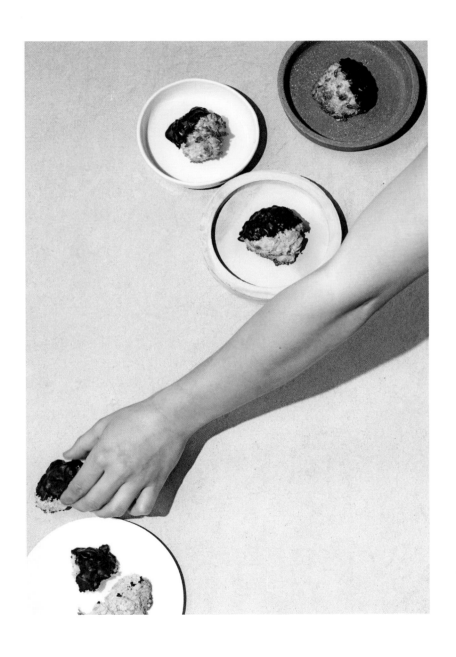

Peanut Butter Chocolate Cake / Salted Caramel

SERVES 6–8

knob of butter, for greasing

300g / 10½oz dark chocolate
(at least 70% cocoa solids),
broken into small pieces

225g / 1¼ cups caster
(superfine) sugar

6 eggs, yolks and whites
separated

225g / 1 cup salted butter,
cut into chunks

2 tsp vanilla extract

175ml / ¾ cup boiling water

5 tbsp GF smooth peanut
butter, loosened with a
splash of boiling water

1 tbsp icing (confectioners')
sugar

SALTED CARAMEL SAUCE

100g / ½ cup caster
(superfine) sugar

30g / 2 tbsp unsalted butter

175ml / ¾ cup single
(light) cream

generous sprinkle of sea salt
flakes

This cake looks wibbly-wobbly and it's meant to. It has a gooey centre and lots of character. Embrace its quirks, or opt for a more refined looking celebration cake on page 144.

Preheat the oven to 180°C / 360°F / gas mark 4. Dot a 26–28cm / 10½–11¼in springform cake tin (pan) with butter and line with parchment paper.

Add the broken chocolate and caster (superfine) sugar to a food processor, and blitz until it turns to fine crumbs. Add the egg yolks, butter, vanilla extract and the boiling water. Blitz again until thoroughly combined.

In a large bowl whisk the egg whites until they form stiff peaks and set to one side.

Pour the chocolate mixture into a separate large bowl and gently fold in the whisked egg whites. Once combined pour the mixture into the lined cake tin, dot in the peanut butter and swirl using a knife. Bake for 45–50 minutes. It's quite a moist cake but should no longer have a wobble to it. It will sink a bit when you take it out of the oven, and is likely to crack a little.

For the salted caramel sauce, add the sugar to a large frying pan and place over a medium heat. Once the sugar has melted, add the butter, stirring the whole time, then add the cream. Once this has turned to caramel add the salt.

Serve the cake warm or cool with the warm sauce. It will also keep really well in the fridge so you can make it a day or two in advance of a dinner party.

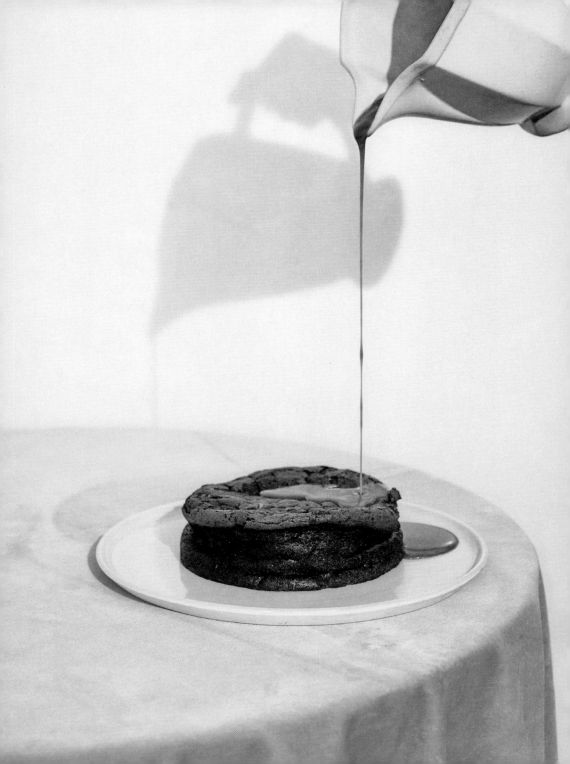

Dutch Baby
/ Caramelized Bananas
& Fresh Orange

SERVES 2

BATTER

180g / 1⅓ cups GF plain
 (all-purpose) flour
¼ tsp baking powder
zest and juice of ½ orange
4 large eggs
150ml / ⅔ cup milk
generous glug of olive oil

BANANAS

3 heaped tbsp golden
 caster (superfine) sugar
 or honey
generous knob of unsalted
 butter
2 bananas, cut in half then
 sliced lengthways

GARNISH

zest of ½ orange, plus flesh
 cut into segments
icing (confectioners') sugar,
 for dusting

First make the Dutch baby. Combine all the batter ingredients except the oil, then place in the fridge to chill for at least 20–30 minutes.

Preheat the oven to 220°C / 425°F / gas mark 7.

Heat a large glug of oil in a cast-iron frying-pan dish over a medium–high heat, then pour in the chilled batter and transfer to the hot oven. Bake for 15–20 minutes until it has risen and turned golden and crisp.

Meanwhile, caramelize the bananas. In a small pan, heat the sugar, allow it to dissolve, then add in the butter, stirring. Once you have a caramel, add in the banana pieces and allow to caramelize. Carefully turn over the banana pieces to cook both sides.

Remove the Dutch baby from the oven.

Spoon the bananas onto the Dutch baby, and add the orange zest and segments. Pour over the caramel sauce and finish with a shake of icing (confectioners') sugar.

Place the pan on the table, and eat while warm.

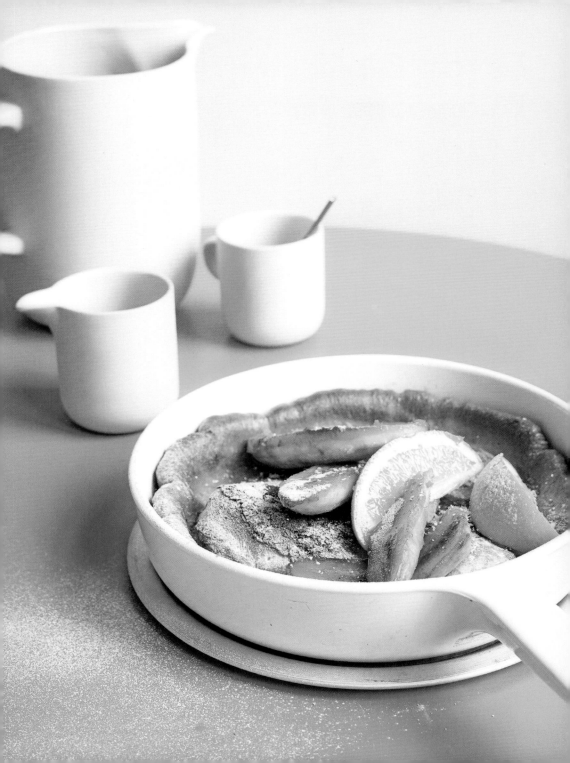

Thyme & Blackberry Frangipane Tart

\\\

**SERVES 6–8 (Makes one
24–26cm / 9½–10½in tart)**

SWEET SHORTCRUST PASTRY

480g / 3⅔ cups GF plain
  (all-purpose) flour, sifted
½ nutmeg, freshly grated
sprinkle of salt
2 heaped tbsp icing
  (confectioners') sugar
220g / 1 cup unsalted butter,
  cubed and chilled
1 egg, beaten
8 sprigs of fresh thyme, leaves
  removed from stalks
3–4 tbsp ice-cold water

FRANGIPANE FILLING

100g / 7 tbsp butter
100g / ½ cup golden caster
  (superfine) sugar, plus
  1 tbsp to sprinkle
2 large eggs
100g / 1 cup ground almonds
370g / 13oz blackberries
5 sprigs of fresh thyme, leaves
  removed from stalks
3 tbsp flaked (slivered)
  almonds

To make the pastry, use a stand mixer and K beater to combine the flour with the nutmeg, salt and icing sugar. Add the butter, combining on a low speed until you have a rough crumb. Add in the egg. When the pastry starts to come together, add the thyme leaves and the ice-cold water, a tablespoon at a time, adding just enough so that the pastry forms into a smooth ball. If you add too much you can add a little extra flour to get the right texture.

Remove the dough from the food processor, roll it out and line a 24–26cm / 9½–10½in tart tin (pan). Prick the pastry all over with a fork and allow to rest in the fridge for around 30 minutes.

Preheat the oven to 180°C / 360°F / gas mark 4. Remove the pastry from the fridge and fill the case with baking beans (or screw up foil and use it to help keep the shape of the tart case). Bake for 15 minutes, remove the baking beans (or foil), then continue to bake for another 5–10 minutes until the pastry is fully cooked – it should be golden brown. Leave the oven on.

To make the filling, beat together the butter and sugar until light and fluffy, then add in the eggs, one at a time, continuing to beat. Gently fold in the almonds and half the blackberries, plus the thyme leaves. Pour the mixture into the cooked pastry case then scatter over the remaining blackberries. Place the tart back into the oven.

When the frangipane has puffed up and is turning golden (after around 35 minutes) scatter over the almonds and sprinkle over the 1 tbsp sugar and cook for a further 4–5 minutes. Remove from the oven and leave to cool a little, before serving warm.

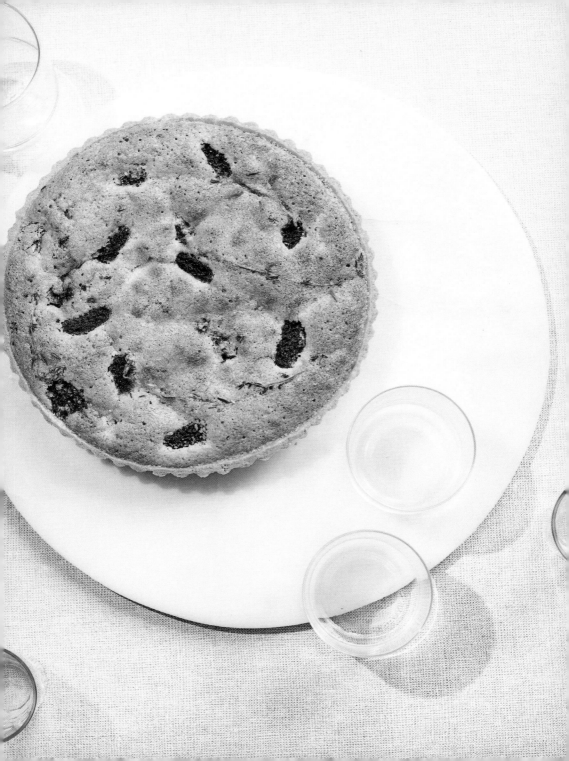

Keep your love of the kitchen alive.

It's easy to despair, throw down your utensils and decide to survive on a diet of ready-made food stuffs. But add kindling to the embers of your passion for cooking by seeking out food surprises and novelties. For example, root out unusual ingredients and unfamiliar fresh produce in international supermarkets; or take the same old veg you normally buy and attack it with kitchen equipment – shave, julienne, ribbon or spiralize to give it (and you) a boost. Try experimenting with flours and baking. And if your lust for food is really deserting you, follow GF food accounts on social media for good-looking inspiration.

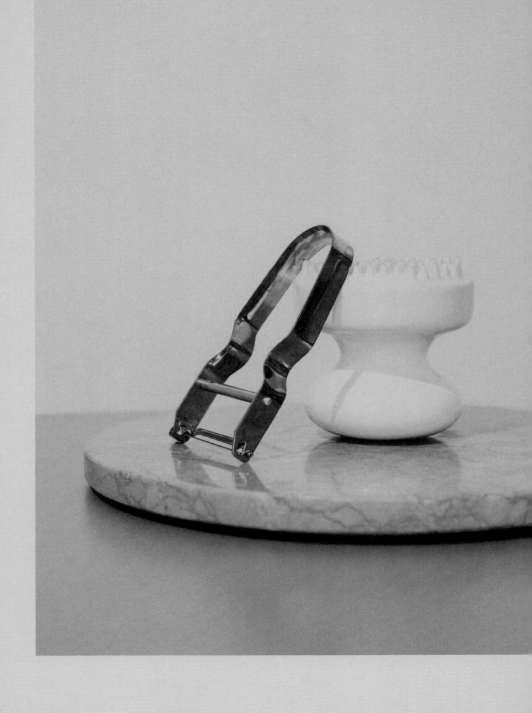

Cardamom & Chocolate Occasion Cake

\\

SERVES 8

300g / 1⅓ cups unsalted
  butter, softened
300g / 1½ cups caster
  (superfine) sugar
4–5 drops of cardamom
  extract
½ tsp vanilla bean paste
4 eggs, beaten
300g / 2¼ cups GF self
  raising (self-rising) flour
90ml / 6 tbsp semi-skimmed
  milk

SALTED CHOCOLATE
BUTTERCREAM

250g / 1 cup plus 2 tbsp
  unsalted butter, softened
550g / scant 4 cups icing
  (confectioners') sugar
4 tbsp cocoa powder
50ml / 3½ tbsp milk
½ tsp sea salt flakes

FROSTING

500g / 2 cup plus 4 tbsp
  unsalted butter, softened
500g / 3½ cups icing
  (confectioners') sugar
800g / 3½ cups cream cheese
pink food colouring

Preheat the oven to 180°C / 360°F / gas mark 4. Line two
16¼–18cm / 6–7in high-sided springform cake tins (pans)
with parchment paper.

Cream together the butter and sugar until light and fluffy.
This can be done by hand or on a low setting in a food
processor or stand mixer. Add the cardamom extract and
vanilla paste to the beaten eggs then add this, a splash at
a time, to the butter and sugar mix until well combined.
Now fold in the flour and milk.

Pour the sponge filling into the lined tins. Weigh
the tins as you pour, so you have equal amounts in
each tin. >>>

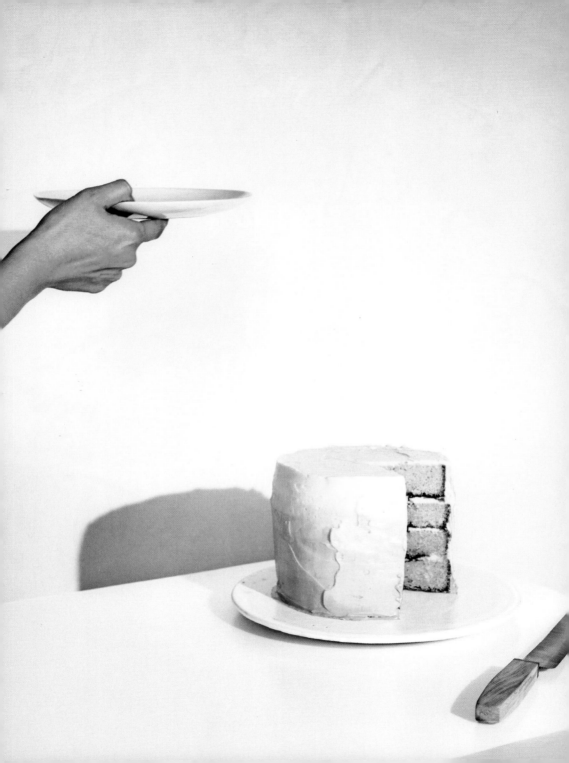

>>> Place the tins in the middle of the oven, side by side, and bake for 20–25 minutes, until they turn golden. To check the sponges are ready, insert a skewer into the middle, no residue should be left on the skewer. Once cooked, turn out onto a wire rack. Once cool, slice each sponge in half horizontally so you have four rounds.

For the salted chocolate buttercream filling, in a food processor or stand mixer, beat the butter until completely soft. Add the icing (confectioners') sugar, cocoa powder and milk, then add the salt. Beat on a high setting for 2–3 minutes, adding in a little more milk for a looser consistency or more icing sugar for a thicker consistency. The filling should hold its shape and not be too sloppy.

For the frosting, combine the butter and icing sugar and beat until combined. Fold in the cream cheese and divide the mixture into four bowls. Add a small amount of pink food colouring to one bowl and combine, making this the darkest shade of pink, then add half the amount of colouring to the next bowl and leave the third and fourth bowls white – one of these will be used as a filling between the layers.

To decorate, place one of the four cake rounds on a serving plate, then spoon on one-third of the white frosting. On top, spoon on one-third of the chocolate buttercream filling, spreading it around, right to the edges. Carefully place the next round on top, and spoon on one-third of the white frosting, and one-third of the remaining

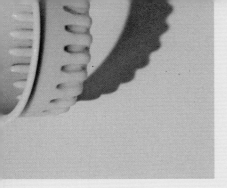

the rest of the filling over it, plus any remaining white
frosting, and then finally add the fourth round to the top.

Using a palette knife or spatula, roughly add a layer of
dark pink frosting around the sides of the cake at the
bottom. Repeat the process with the pale pink frosting,
making a layer that sits just above the dark pink and
repeat once more with the white frosting, covering the
top also.

Now take your spatula and blend the layers, working
round the cake so the dark pink and pale pink are now
blended a little and the pale pink and white are also
blended where they meet. Chill or serve immediately.

Rose Panna Cotta / Burnt Orange

MAKES 4

100ml / generous ⅓ cup milk

400ml / 1¾ cups double (heavy) cream

2 vanilla pods

1½ sheets gelatine

50g / ⅓ cup icing (confectioners') sugar

2 tsp rose water

GARNISH

juice of 1 blood orange or orange

caster (superfine) sugar, for sprinkling

1 orange, peeled and thinly sliced

Pour the milk and about two-thirds of the cream into a small saucepan. Cut the vanilla pods in half, scrape out the seeds with a knife and add both the seeds and pods to the cream. Simmer gently for 5–6 minutes.

Soak the gelatine sheets in a bowl of cold water. After 5 minutes or so the gelatine will soften. Gently beat the remaining cream with the icing (confectioners') sugar.

Remove the cream from the heat, add the rose water and lift out the vanilla pods. Stir in the sheets of softened gelatine until dissolved, then fold in the sweetened cream.

Pour through a sieve (strainer) then transfer the mixture into four moulds and leave to cool. Cover and refrigerate until set (this will take about 2–3 hours).

Combine the orange juice and caster sugar in a small pan and reduce a little over a medium–high heat until it becomes a little syrup-like.

Remove the chilled panna cottas from the fridge and turn out onto serving plates. If they stick, soak them in a bowl of boiling water for a few seconds to loosen them.

Soak the orange slices in the juice, then drizzle a little of the juice over each of the panna cottas. Place an orange round on top of each panna cotta, then spoon on a little caster (superfine) sugar and heat with a blow torch until slightly blackened.

Rich Chocolate Orange Pots / Nut Brittle

SERVES 6–8

280ml / 1¼ cups double (heavy) cream

1 tbsp caster (superfine) sugar

40g / 3 tbsp unsalted butter

200g / 7oz dark chocolate (at least 70% cocoa solids), broken into small pieces

50ml / 3½ tbsp full-fat milk

sprinkle of sea salt flakes

zest of 1 orange

juice of ½ orange

2 tbsp orange liqueur

fresh orange segments, to serve (optional)

NUT BRITTLE

280g / 1½ cups caster (superfine) sugar

120g / 4oz nuts of your choice

sea salt flakes, for sprinkling

To make the chocolate orange pots, first heat the cream and sugar together in a small pan until almost boiling. Remove from the heat and add the butter and chocolate, stirring until you have a smooth consistency.

Next add the milk, stirring again, then add the sea salt, orange zest and juice, and orange liqueur. Stir until you have a smooth, glossy consistency then divide between 6–8 serving cups or glasses (or pour into one large serving bowl) and allow to cool. Transfer to the fridge to set once cooled. It will take around 1–2 hours.

To make the brittle, lightly toast the nuts for 2–3 minutes in a dry saucepan, then transfer to a sealable container and give it a good shake, removing the skin from the nuts as best you can. Roughly chop the nuts and set to one side.

Line two large baking trays (pans) with parchment paper.

Add the sugar to a dry saucepan and place over a low heat, letting it form clumps and eventually turn to a medium then dark caramel. When it does, remove the pan from the heat, add in the chopped nuts and mix before pouring out onto the parchment-lined trays. Sprinkle with salt flakes.

To make an extra-thin brittle, cover the hot caramel with another sheet of parchment and use a rolling pin to roll it to your preferred thickness. Allow to cool for around 10–15 minutes, break into shards, then store in an airtight container until ready to serve.

Serve the chocolate pots with orange segments or just with shards of the nut brittle.

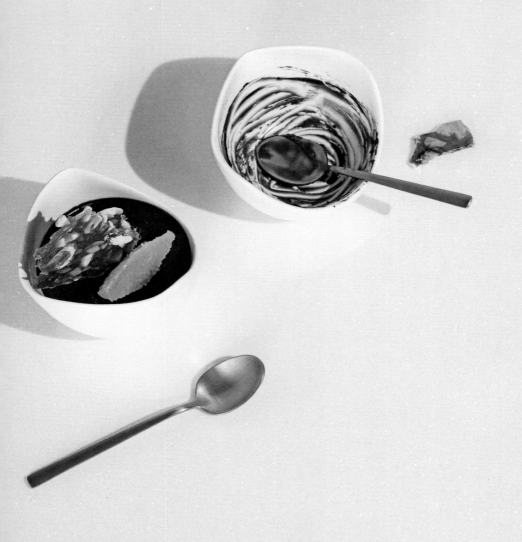

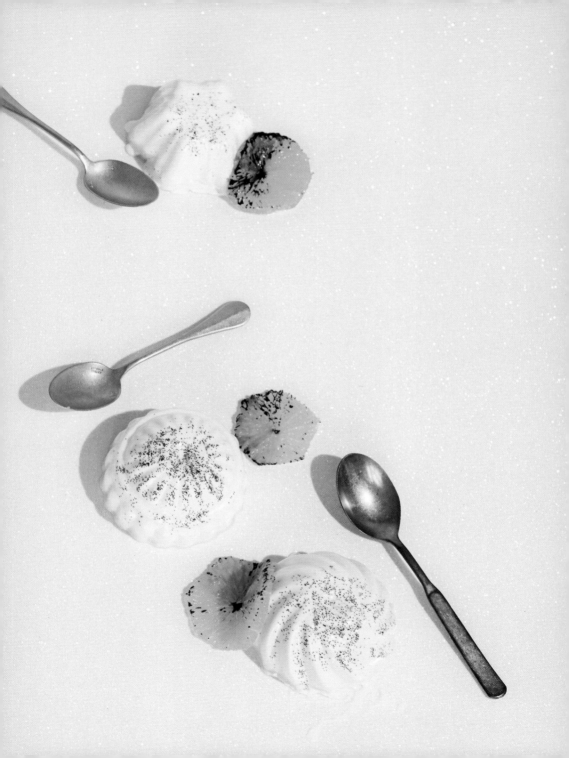

Gin & Pink Tonic Ice Pops

MAKES 6–8

100ml / 6–7 tbsp gin
320ml / 1¼ cup pink or regular tonic
zest of 1 lime
juice of 2 limes
6–8 kaffir lime leaves

Combine the gin, tonic and the lime zest and juice in a jug (pitcher).

Place a kaffir lime leaf in each ice pop mould and pour over the mixture. (If using wooden lolly sticks, position them now.) Place the pops in the freezer for 2–3 hours.

Serve when frozen.

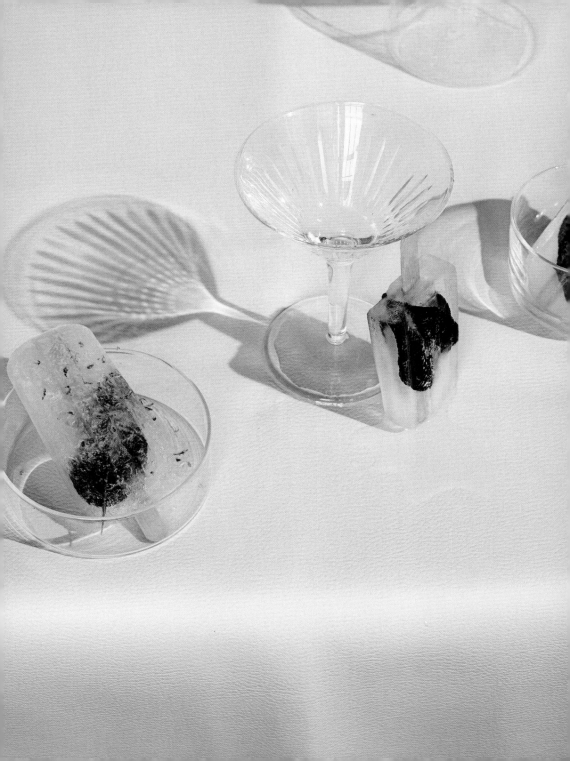

Find a friend.

It can get tedious constantly explaining your dietary requirements or hunting out gluten-free food, which is why it's good to find an ally. It can be someone that's already in your life, or someone who you meet through a GF society. But we all need that person who has our back: someone who is happy to negotiate with the restaurant wait staff on our behalf, or get excited about a new GF brownie recipe from heaven. Know who's on your side, stick with them, and appreciate them.

Find peace.

Troublesome gluten isn't going to go away. But life can be brilliant, full of amazing food, night's out and friends who barely register your 'special' diet. To reach this GF nirvana, you need to find your inner grit and nurture it, then use it to navigate the trials and pitfalls of GF living with grace and optimism. It won't always be plain sailing, but learn to ride the waves and you will find a more zen gluten-free life just around the corner...

\\\

Publishing Director Sarah Lavelle
Commissioning Editor Zena Alkayat
Design Manager Claire Rochford
Art Direction / Design Maeve Bargman
Cover Design Luke Bird
Photographer Kim Lightbody
Props Stylist Rachel Vere
Recipe Writer and Food Stylist Anna Barnett
Food Stylist's Assistant Hannah Miller
Production Director Vincent Smith
Production Controller Nikolaus Ginelli

Published in 2018 by Quadrille,
an imprint of Hardie Grant Publishing

Reprinted in 2019, 2020
10 9 8 7 6 5 4

Quadrille
52–54 Southwark Street
London SE1 1UN
quadrille.com

ISBN 978 1 78713 291 7

Printed in China